Doctors as Managers

Experiences in the front-line of the NHS

Editors

Roger Hadley and Don Forster

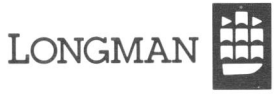

LONGMAN

Longman Group UK Limited
Westgate House, The High, Harlow, Essex CM20 1YR
Telephone (0279) 442601
Fax (0279) 444501

First published 1993

A catalogue record for this book is available from the British Library.

ISBN 0-582-22861-1

Printed in Great Britain by Redwood Books, Trowbridge, Wiltshire

For

Clare Wenger and Chris Forster

Contents

Preface

The ultimate test of the quality of a health care organisation, whether for patient or doctor, is the nature of the service provided by its front-line units. Yet the subject of how these units are actually managed in practice, and what makes for effective or ineffective leadership at this level, whether in ward, clinic, or surgery, is curiously neglected. Reams have been written on technical and financial management as they apply at almost every rung in the NHS hierarchy, but the nitty-gritty of the human dynamics of the organisation at the point where it meets its users has attracted little systematic analysis whether by academics or practitioners.

We suspect that this neglect owes more to the inaccessibility of the subject than a lack of interest in it or a rejection of its importance. Quite properly, those running health service organisations are concerned to protect patients' right to confidentiality and to be cautious about allowing researchers access to the front-line settings where treatment is carried out. Less disinterestedly, they may not relish the upheaval and challenge that close scrutiny of team management can create, and the panoply of profession and hierarchy make it relatively easy to block unwelcome investigators. However, it would also seem that some doctors, at least until very recently, have failed to see front-line management as even being a relevant issue: expertise dictates procedures, the senior doctor as the most expert member of the team expects and receives the compliance of its other members. In this context, team management, at the most, is a matter of telling other people what to do and requires neither research nor training to carry out successfully.

This book bypasses such barriers to front-line units by presenting accounts of their management, not by researchers or other outside observers, but by doctors who have been junior members of front-line teams themselves. While their case studies are based on personal experience rather than systematic research, they are more than merely anecdotal. All were written in the context of a course on organisational behaviour and all seek to apply concepts developed in the course. The special interest of the ten case studies involved is, therefore, of two kinds. Firstly, for what they reveal about the nature of management in the front-line units in the NHS; secondly, for what they imply about the contribution of an enhanced understanding of organisational behaviour in improving it. Their reports and reflections on the former are sufficiently critical and disturbing to emphasise the considerable importance of the latter.

Of course, the small sample of cases presented in this book can in no way claim to be representative of such a large organisation as the NHS. We hope, nevertheless, that it may at least serve the purposes of stimulating more systematic and extensive work in this area, and of encouraging a wider debate on the importance of training doctors as managers, not only of financial and technical resources, but also of human beings.

We are indebted to and gratefully thank the contributors of the case studies for the perceptive and thoughtful accounts of their experiences of medical organisations which constitute the core of the book. For obvious reasons, it was decided that the contributors should remain anonymous. Similarly, the settings in which they worked have not been identified and aspects of these have been altered, although not in ways which have compromised the contributors' analyses.

We also acknowledge the most helpful contributions of Karen Cowley and Sandra Irving in the preparation of the manuscript, of Richard Hadley in preparing final versions of the diagrams on pages 14, 48, 50, 66, 96, 105, 108, 114, 118, 127, 128, 132 and of Professor Clare Wenger in commenting on drafts of the editorial sections of the book.

Roger Hadley and *Don Forster*
February 1993

Glossary

This glossary gives a brief explanation of technical terms used in the case studies. Where appropriate, the reader is also referred to the section of the Introduction where the topic concerned is placed in context and where references to the relevant literature can also be found.

Action perspective
This approach emphasises that while people are defined by the society they live in, they also in turn define that society, modifying and changing social meanings. In organisational analysis it encourages an emphasis on an understanding which includes the perspective of all the participants, not simply those in positions of formal authority (page 289).

Authority
In organisations legitimate power is based on position or expertise or both (pages 23–4).

Benevolent authoritative management (System 2)
Leadership characterised by master–servant like trust, motivation based on a mix of reward and punishment, no involvement in decisions but occasional consultation (page 27).

Bureaucracy
Literally, government by officials. In organisation theory, the use of the term is strongly influenced by Max Weber's definition as the form of organisation associated with legal-rational authority. Emphasis on hierarchy, the division of labour, rules, appointment and promotion on basis of proved skills. (See page 22.)

Consultative management (System 3)
Leadership founded on a considerable measure of confidence in subordinates, motivation mainly based on rewards but some punishment, employees usually consulted about work decisions but do not share in them (page 27).

Contingency theory
Theory that there is no one best way to structure and manage organisations and that different approaches are required according to task, environment, and other factors involved (pages 21–3).

Dominant coalition
A group whose members between them share the effective control of an organisation or unit. They may or may not coincide with those who hold the formal authority to wield this control (page 24).

Exploitive authoritative management (System 1)
Leadership based on direction, absence of trust of subordinates, motivation by fear, close supervision, no consultation about work decisions (page 27).

Human relations theory
Based on the view that people's needs in organisations are seldom satisfied by the formal structure and that they look for a sense of belonging and significance in their work. *Neo-human relations theory* has extended this approach by broadening the concept of needs to include personal development and self-actualisation and defining the kinds of organisational structure in which this might be achieved (pages 26–7).

Involvement
The nature of people's commitment to an organisation. One simple but valuable classification distinguishes between alienative (negative), moral (positive, identifying with norms of the organisation) and calculative (or instrumental) involvement (page 28).

Lower participants
People at lower levels in the hierarchy of an organisation. The term has been used in conjunction with studies of power in organisations to show that people at these levels may sometimes have access to more power and influence than their formal position would imply (pages 23–4).

Maintenance activities
Term used in socio-technical systems analysis to describe activities which supply the resources needed by an organisation's operating activities, such as equipment, personnel, training, and motivation of employees.

Mission task
Goal(s) of an organisation other than that (those) required to ensure its survival (primary task, q.v.). Should be distinguished from popular contemporary use of the term to describe, usually for public consumption, the overall goals of an organisation (page 25).

Negotiated order
A view that at any one time the social structure of an organisation is determined not simply by the formal roles and tasks of its members, but also by complex inter-personal bargaining and negotiation (pages 28–9).

Operating activities
Term used in socio-technical systems analysis to describe the activities in an organisation which directly contribute to the input, conversion, and output processes which define the primary task of the organisation.

Participative management (System 4)
Leadership based on complete trust of subordinates, reward system determined through group participation, organisational decisions widely shared, employees fully involved in work-related decisions (page 27).

Primary task
Term used to describe the activities which an organisation must carry out successfully in order to survive (page 25).

Power
The ability of person or group to gain the compliance or obedience of others to his/her/their will. In organisational studies *power* is contrasted with *authority* (q.v.). Various sources of such power can be identified apart from official position in an organisation including expertise, control of resources, personal qualities, coercion, and the ability to withold coopera-tion sometimes referred to as negative power (page 23–4).

Regulatory activities
Term used in socio-technical systems analysis to describe activities which relate to each other the operating and maintenance activities, and all internal sub-systems, and also to relate the organisation to its environment (page 25).

Scientific management
Theory associated with the work of F. W. Taylor based on the view that the 'one best way' of carrying out any task can be scientifically established and that organisational structures and processes should be designed by managers in the light of this (page 20).

Sentient group
Term used by some socio-technical systems researchers to describe groups with which people identify themselves and feel loyalty to, as opposed to task groups determined by the organisation and for which they may or may not have such feelings (page 25).

Systems theory
Management versions draw on basic notions which see systems as a group of elements related together in an organised way to achieve a particular purpose or purposes. *Open systems* approaches see organisations, much as biological organisms, existing by exchanging materials with their environ-ment through a process of input-conversion-output (pages 24–6).

Systems 1, 2, 3, and 4
See exploitive authoritative, benevolent authoritative, consultative and participative management.

Theory X
Average human beings inherently dislike work, need as a result to be coerced, directed, threatened with punishment to get them to work, and prefer to be directed and avoid taking responsibility. Security is their prime aim (pages 26–7).

Theory Y
For average human beings, work is as natural as rest and play, they can be self-directing when committed to the objectives served, learn to accept and seek responsibility, and have the potential to use imagination, ingenuity and creativity in the solution of organisational problems (pages 26–7).

List of Abbreviations

A & E	Accident and Emergency
CMO	Clinical Medical Officer
CO	Clerical Officer
DGH	District General Hospital
DHA	District Health Authority
DHSS	Department of Health and Social Security
DMT	District Management Team
DOH	Department of Health
EC	Executive Council
FHSA	Family Health Service Authority
FPC	Family Practitioner Committee
GAA	General Administrative Assistant
GNP	Gross National Product
GP	General Practitioner
GPT	General Professional Training
GYNAE	Gynaecology
HCO	Higher Clerical Officer
HO	House Officer
JCHMT	Joint Committee for Higher Medical Training
MRCP	Member of the Royal College of Physicians
NHS	National Health Service
NO	Nursing Officer
OP	Outpatients
OR	Operational Research
PHCT	Primary Health Care Team
R or REG	Registrar
RHA	Regional Health Authority
SCMO	Senior Clinical Medical Officer
SEN	State Enrolled Nurse
SHO	Senior House Officer
SNO	Senior Nursing Officer
SR	Senior Registrar
SRN	State Registered Nurse

PART I

Introduction

Introduction

The case for a consideration of organisational matters in the health care sector is compelling. In the developed countries of the world, some 6 per cent to 12 per cent of Gross National Product is expended on health care in the public or private sector. Moreover, for the most part health care organisations provide personal health care by individuals and hence are highly labour intensive. In Britain, the National Health Service (NHS) employs in excess of one million persons and is one of the largest employers in Europe. In volume terms alone, therefore, health care ranks alongside the largest industrial and commercial enterprises.

In contrast to the industrial and commercial sector, however, where the inputs, processes and outputs are often highly standardised, the patients who enter health care are infinitely variable and the challenges to management are peculiarly complex. The diagnostic and therapeutic processes which patients undergo are not only personal but frequently at hospital level involve the use of high technology. Given this necessary use of both people skills and clinical technical skills by health care personnel, the measurement of the quality of processes and outcomes of health care is particularly difficult. A further complicating factor for understanding these organisations in Britain, where the largest part of their work is concentrated in the public sector, is that their funding relies mainly on direct support from the state. The introduction of a limited internal market within the public sector is only serving to add still greater complexity to the task of those managing them. The challenge of managing health care organisations is further compounded by their tendency to have multiple functions. For example, although their first task is almost invariably the provision of health care, teaching and research are frequently found as additional activities. Moreover, in contrast to more traditional organisations where professionals are typically employed as advisers and seldom have much direct management authority, in most health care organisations the front-line work is often managed and carried out by well educated, skilled, and in some instances highly paid professionals. In other words, in these organisations the professionals – and especially the doctors – often have power and authority to match their status.

In sum, health care organisations in general and the NHS in particular pose special challenges to those who plan and manage them. A good

1

understanding of their special characteristics as organisations is a pre-requisite of their effective and efficient management. Further, this understanding needs to embrace not only macro issues which affect the organisations as a whole but to recognise the central importance of front-line units in health care and to include the micro level as well.

Front-line management in the NHS

Given the importance of health care in national economies (in addition to the self-evident importance for individual patients) and the complex position of professionals in the organisation, it might be expected that the relationship between the changes that have taken place in the NHS since its inception and organisational or managerial theory would have been the subject of intensive discussion and research. This has not proved to be the case since the bulk of the contributions have tended to concentrate on structural changes to the NHS and technical developments such as planning, costs in relationship to benefits, and the audit of quality and performance (as examples: *Accounting for health, 1973*; Levitt & Wall, 1984; Ham, 1991). The behavioural aspects of these technical processes have been relatively neglected (Cox, 1991).

However, the pace of change required in the NHS, dictated partly through advances in clinical medicine but predominantly through government-induced change in a politically governed service, necessitates and adds further to the case for seeking to enhance our understanding of behavioural factors in organisational performance. In spite of this, it could be said that in the past compliance with change seems often to have been taken as non-problematical and the organisation and management element in the training of key professionals is still relatively small. Indeed, such training is almost non-existent at undergraduate medical student levels, in which it tends to be crowded out of an already overstretched curriculum by the powerful demands of the clinical specialties. At postgraduate level, the need for managerial training is recognised but its provision is haphazard rather than systematic. It is still possible for a clinician to face significant managerial tasks for the first time after appointment as a consultant without extensive prior training.

Although the NHS is moving from a system of planned health care to one in which decision making is to be responsive to market mechanisms, most management interactions continue to involve doctors and frequently doctors as managers. Indeed, with the growing emphasis on devolving responsibilities within the health service closer to the front-line, whether in the hospital or in the budget-holding general practice, the managerial role of doctors is likely to become even more significant. It remains an open question to what extent this role will be shaped by the increasing power and influence of non-medical managers. As a recent commentator on current changes in the NHS has noted 'Retrenchment, restructuring, and market reforms have at the same time enabled and legitimated health-service managerialism, and a systematic reduction in professional medical autonomy' (Flynn, 1992, p.196). Yet, as the same writer acknowledges, 'it is unlikely that medical dominance in the division of labour and policy-making will be completely undermined' by this development (Ibid, p.196). The very nature of professional work and the exercise of discretion which it involves, requires at least a modicum of autonomy if it is to be effective. Beyond this, however, the extent to which doctors can deflect or modify the pressures brought to bear on them and retain a significant degree of control over their work may well be affected by their ability to become effective managers of their own front-line units. This, in turn, we would argue, will depend on their ability to develop a good understanding of these units and their functioning in behavioural as well as in technical and clinical terms.

This book seeks to make a contribution to broadening the debate on front-line management in the NHS by focusing on the practical experience of a number of doctor-participants in different parts of the service. The Case Studies contributed by these participants were written during their training in public health medicine. All the studies are centrally concerned with behavioural aspects of management and provide the data on which the three central themes which inform this book are based:

– The nature and significance of front-line management in doctor-led units
– The potential contribution of organisational analysis in developing an understanding of the dynamics of such management
– The role of experiential learning in acquiring the skills of organisational analysis and improving management practice

The importance of front-line management as a key determinant of the effectiveness of the services provided for patients is not the central focus of this book but, nevertheless, is illustrated directly or indirectly in each of the case studies.

The book is divided into three main sections. In the introduction we provide the context for the doctors' Case Studies, firstly outlining the formal structures of the NHS within which the organisations studied were located; secondly, setting behavioural approaches in the broader framework of perspectives more typically used in health service evaluation; and finally, sketching the main aspects of organisational theory on which the contributors have drawn in their analyses. The second part of the book contains the ten critical Case Studies of the management of doctor-led front-line units in different parts of the NHS. These are grouped in terms of the three themes of equilibrium, conflict and change. In the conclusions we review common elements in the Case Studies, consider the value of theory in enhancing our understanding of the organisations studied, and outline a suggested check-list for front-line managers who may want to apply a similar approach to the analysis of their own work settings. Finally, we examine wider issues in the selection and training of doctors as managers which emerge from the case studies.

The context of NHS organisation

In this section we describe the wider context for the Case Studies contained in this book. First, for those unfamiliar with the history of the NHS, we offer a short sketch of its evolution, concentrating mainly on the last two decades. This is followed by a more narrowly focused discussion of the role of doctors in front-line management, including the parts played by the clinical firm and the nature of the medical career structure.

Origins and development of the health service

The origins and development of the front-line units of medical practice analysed later in the Case Studies can be traced back to the eighteenth and nineteenth centuries. Then, the forerunners of general practitioners were the apothecaries who mainly worked single handed from their own homes (Fry, 1988). Their rivals for patients, particularly in London, were the physicians and surgeons. Physicians and surgeons, who were of higher status than apothecaries, gave their services free to charitable or voluntary hospitals but charged fees to their private patients in the community. The competition for fee paying patients in the community was resolved by the acceptance in the professions of the referral system through which apothecaries were excluded from the hospitals, but referred their patients to the physicians and surgeons for more specialised consultations. The result of this development was that physicians and surgeons did not compete directly with the apothecaries for patients in the community, but the two arms of the profession became dependent on one another (British Medical Association, 1970). This interdependence, yet separation, of generalist practice and practitioners in the community from the more specialised practice in hospitals continues to this day.

In the first four decades of this century, before the Second World War, the health services in Britain had a tripartite structure. The general practitioner was the first point of contact for the ill in the community, although most dependents of those working were still not covered by the national health insurance scheme. Acute hospital care was provided largely in the voluntary hospitals and longer-term care in local authority or municipal hospitals. Preventive health care was the concern of the local authorities. During the war years, the formation of the Emergency Medical Service brought together the voluntary and local authority hospitals under a single national and regional administration for the first time (Fry, 1988).

Proposals for a national health service that would integrate the separate elements of provision and create a universal system of care in the country took shape in the 1920s and 1930s but only became the focus of national debate during the Second World War (Willcocks, 1967). The Beveridge Report (Beveridge, 1942) insisted that a national health service was an essential underpinning for an effective reconstruction of the system of social security, a view shared by the incoming Labour Government in 1945. The NHS bill was introduced in 1946 (National Health Service Bill, 1946) and the new service was implemented in 1948. The tripartite structure of health services between the hospitals, general practice and local authorities was maintained in the new NHS. In the early years of austerity that followed the end of the war there was relatively little development in the new service. Work tended to be concentrated on administering what was present rather than effecting change. Committees for the appointment of consultants to hospitals were comprised mostly of doctors and therefore helped to perpetuate the prevailing values of professional autonomy. As clinical firms enlarged, there was, however, a movement towards the designation of one consultant as the consultant in administrative charge of the provision of particular clinical services. Such appointments were often based on seniority rather than some assessment of management skills.

This is not to say that there were no significant management developments before the first major reorganisation of the NHS in 1974. Three working parties on the organisation of medical work in hospitals (known as the Cogwheel Reports) recommended that clinical specialties of a similar nature should be amalgamated into divisions, and meetings held involving both senior and junior medical staff (Ministry of Health, 1967; DHSS, 1972; DHSS, 1974). The function of each division was to review the provision and use of clinical services under its remit. The representatives of each division were to meet as a medical executive committee, whose chairman would represent the view of all the hospital clinical staff and liaise with the nursing staff and administration. In the context of a book focusing on front-line management, it is interesting to note that the emphasis in the management issues covered by the Cogwheel reports was primarily on the efficiency of use of resources, and that the styles or skills of management which can be so important in achieving such efficiency were ignored.

There were also moves to improve management in nursing during this period. The Salmon Report reviewed and made recommendations on the nursing management structure (Ministry of Health and Scottish Home and Health Department, 1966), which were subsequently adopted. These recommendations formalised existing nursing hierarchies by creating the grades of chief, principal, senior and nursing officers. The implementation of Salmon gave nursing and its management greater autonomy from doctors but was not without its problems. Decisions at ward level, usually generated by doctors but in conjunction with the ward sister, were now complicated by the presence of higher tiers of nursing management. Additionally, in order to progress beyond ward sister or charge nurse level, a nurse had to leave the clinical sphere of work. Many doctors and nurses saw the resulting loss of the most experienced and skilled nursing staff from the front-line as a high price to pay for improved management.

The 1974 reorganisation

The primary purpose of the reorganisation of 1974 was to unify the tripartite structure of the NHS into a single integrated organisation (*National Health Service Reorganisation: England*, 1972). The previously separate organisation of the hospital system, general practice, and community and public health services made liaison in patient care and management difficult to achieve and had created a structure resistant to overall planning. In brief, the services brought together under the broad umbrella of a single organisation included hospital services, general practitioner services (plus general dental, opthalmic and pharmaceutical services) and health services previously run by local authorities (eg health visiting, district nursing, community midwifery, well baby and child development clinics, vaccination and immunisation, school health services and ambulance services). Some health-related services still remained outside the NHS: for instance personal social services (including hospital social work) remained a function and responsibility of local authorities (Office of Health Economics, 1974).

The fundamental entity of the new organisation was the health district. These covered populations of about 250,000 persons, on average, not necessarily conterminous with local authorities, but containing a District General Hospital (DGH) catering for the main specialties. The management team at district level comprised four officers, the district nursing officer, the district community physician, the finance officer and district administrator. In addition, the team included two clinicians, namely the chairman and vice chairman of the District Medical Committee, a hospital consultant and a GP elected through the Cogwheel advisory mechanisms. As public watchdogs, Community Health Councils were set up as bodies separate from the District Management Team (DMT) but with rights of access to plans. Although higher levels of management authorities were also established, for example statutory Area Health Authorities coterminous with metropolitan local authority districts or non-metropolitan counties and Regional Health Authorities (RHAs) (replacing Regional Hospital Boards), the district became the focus for the development and implementation of plans within guidelines from above. Family Practitioner Committees (FPCs), coterminous with Area Health Authorities, replaced Executive Councils, but were little changed. They continued to administer services for GPs and others as independent contractors to the NHS with direct links to the Department of Health and Social Services (DHSS).

The essence of decision making at District Management Team (DMT) level (and higher levels in the NHS) was one of consensus. However, decision making and the implementation of decisions through this semblance of participation was impeded by a number of factors. Firstly, the job descriptions and roles of the district officers on the DMT were tightly drawn, a reminder of the influence of Taylorism on the advisers to the management arrangements. Unfortunately, this prescription of 'scientifically trained' individuals for particular roles was not accompanied by any motivating influences. Secondly, the clinicians on the team, although described as delegates, were really representatives of the clinician body and could not necessarily count on their colleagues to deliver what had been agreed. Moreover, it was frequently clinicians from the more powerful specialties who had access to the DMT and thus controlled the agenda for action (Haywood & Alaszewski, 1980).

In 1982, a further reorganisation recognised the overlap and conflict between decision-making at district and area level. The outcome was to abandon the area tier of management, the district now became the statutory health authority with direct links to the regional health authority. The geographical coterminosity, for the coordinated planning of hospital and community services with local authority provided services, was consequently lost except in metropolitan districts.

The introduction of general management

What can now be seen as a much more important development followed a year later with the publication of the Griffiths Report on NHS management (DHSS, 1983). Griffiths' highly critical document noted that there was a lack of direction, drive, speed and responsibility in decision making in the existing consensus process. His main proposals included the setting up of a Supervisory Board within the DHSS to determine strategy and an NHS Management Board, accountable to the former, to implement approved policies. At regional, district and hospital (unit) levels, a general manager was to be appointed to have overall responsibility for achieving the objectives of the relevant health authority. Decisions concerning all functions in the organisation would therefore be vested in the general manager. Griffiths proposed that clinicians should be drawn closely into

7

the management process and suggested that the Cogwheel procedures provided a basis for this.

In the following years, as the recommendations of the report were implemented, it was felt by some that clinical freedom had been underestimated by Griffiths and subsequent BMA debates frequently contained allegations that health managers were undermining this freedom (Dyson, 1984; the *Guardian*, 1987). There was, however, a dichotomy of opinion in that some clinicians welcomed taking on the general management function and saw that there would be no shortage of candidates from other professions if doctors rejected this role (Hopkins, 1987). In practice, doctors formally combined clinical and managerial roles most frequently as clinical or specialty directors. In this position, they were responsible to the general manager of the hospital for the service provided by the specialty. Frequently, they had the support of a specialty business manager and liaised with clinical colleagues (over whom there was no formal authority), nursing managers and other professions involved in providing the overall specialty service (Mumford, 1989).

Injecting market ideology

In 1989, while the changes in management introduced following the Griffiths Report were still being digested, the NHS Review proposed the most radical organisational change in health care since the inception of the service itself in 1948 (Secretaries of State for Health, Wales, Northern Ireland and Scotland, 1989). The ideology behind the changes involved the introduction of the principles of the private sector and the market into the publicly financed system (Forster & Hadley, 1989). The practical changes supporting this philosophy included the separation of health authorities as purchasers, from hospitals as providers, the majority of which were to be encouraged to become self-governing trusts independent of health authority control. Certain selected larger general practices (budget-holding practices) also had the option of becoming purchasers of hospital services on behalf of their patients.

The management of clinical activity in the new arrangements is governed, therefore, through the contractual process for clinical services between purchasers and providers. The general management function, and the involvement of clinicians as clinical directors, is therefore, considerably reinforced by these changes (Ham, 1991). Concomitant changes in the GP contract also relate payments more closely to the achievement of certain activities, for instance the running of prevention clinics or routine assessments of the elderly (Department of Health and the Welsh Office, 1989).

The Supervisory Board in the Department of Health and the NHS Management Board are retained, but renamed the Policy Board and

Management Executive respectively. Regional Health Authorities and District Health Authorities were maintained and Family Practitioner Committees renamed as Family Health Service Authorities. The representative nature of the membership of these authorities has, however, been drastically curtailed. Membership of each of the small business-orientated authorities consists of a chairman appointed by the Secretary of State for Health, officers of the authority itself, including the chief executive, and non-executive members appointed to each authority by the RHA. It can be readily appreciated that these procedures potentially support the placement of members in a health authority who have the 'correct' ideological views.

The way in which the Conservative government enacted change in the NHS, based on their 1989 proposals, is worth considering. The values underlying the government's motivation for change were ostensibly based on a perceived lack of patient choice and wide variations in service performance in different parts of the country, such as the costs of treating acute hospital patients and GP drug prescription costs. The proposals introduced tension into the system through the creation and maintenance of a sense of uncertainty for NHS staff about the funding for their hospital or unit. This situation may be exacerbated for employees through probable increased use of short-term employment contracts by Trusts in the future thus strengthening the hand of managers. In brief, the government's case for change rested on its dissatisfaction with the absence of market forces in the system, yet the main professional groups expressed their dissatisfactions mainly in terms of the underfunding of the NHS rather than as faults in its structure and operation. General managers were the group most willing to engage in the process of change whereas the professional groups were the resisters.

In attempting to unfreeze resistance to change, the government gave weight and influence to its, arguably dubious, negative evaluation of the present organisation of the NHS and its higher expectations for the future (Forster & Hadley, 1989). By and large, it rejected other well tried methods of unfreezing resistance, for example open discussion and negotiation and piloting of the changes. The NHS Review itself was carried out 'in camera', rather than in the public forum of a Royal Commission or committee of inquiry, and the implementation was the sole test of the viability of the ideas expressed in the review. Although the government has had the authority and power to impose the formal changes that it defined in the review, other conditions necessary for successful movement and 'refreezing' in the change process have only been partially met. If changes in an organisation are to 'stick', it is insufficient that the objectives alone should be clear. The self esteem of the participants needs to be raised and externally provided motives for change need to be replaced by internalised motives (Dalton et al, 1968). We noted above that the management of clinical activity was bound up with the issue of contracts. The involvement of clinicians in this process implies a change from previously cooperative professional values to business relationships. Current evidence suggests that the management–clinician partnership under the new market system may not have been as successful as the government anticipated as health authorities run out of money for clinical service contracts in the final quarter of 1992/93. This has again caused the medical profession to express concern about underfunding (Dillner, 1993).

The neglect of the front-line unit

From this brief review of the changes that have taken place in the organisation of health services, it can be seen that the recommendations for organisational revision have been concentrated at the macro level, usually that at the hospital or above. The drive for change has been derived until recently from a desire for comprehensiveness and coordination within a single service, with clear lines of communication and management. The other motivation which has increasingly been to the fore in the reorganisations of the NHS has been that of efficiency, even though the tools available for its measurement are rudimentary. What each organisational revision has failed to address is how the detailed logistics of management of the front-line units which actually deliver the service, may be affected. This gap in official thinking is particularly marked in respect of the behavioural elements of the operation of these units. Yet, as the whole history of formal organisations amply demonstrates, the level of motivation and active cooperation of the producers of a service are of the essence in determining its efficiency and effectiveness. Given this lack of attention to, and involvement in, the decisions about change, some would say that it is surprising how well the workforce of the NHS has responded to the frequent modifications to its structure and processes. Alternatively, however, it could be argued that in reality the changes have yet to make any major impact on the management of the front-line units. Instead, these continue to be run in ways which have more to do with tradition and the idiosyncracies of their particular managers than the formal ideologies and principles which are officially supposed to drive the service. These are questions which can be considered further in the case studies of front-line units presented in this book.

The role and influence of doctors in management

Before the NHS came into being, it was common for hospitals to have a physician superintendent who derived power from both medical and executive roles. Although some physician superintendents continued in this position after the inception of the NHS, especially in psychiatric hospitals, executive authority became the province of the administrators of the newly created Hospital Boards. The power of doctors in the early NHS years rested, therefore, not on formal roles but on their pivotal position in front-line care. This involved not only a key place in decisions about the delivery of treatment and care to individual patients and the possession of professional skills to enact that care, but also implied control over the resources required. The professional expertise of doctors dominated the agenda for action within the NHS (Haywood & Alaszewski, 1980) at local levels and was more tangibly recognised in the professional advisory structures set up at local, regional and national levels.

Origins of the clinical firm

The referral process, negotiated much earlier between apothecaries (GPs) and hospital consultants confined specialist care and treatments to hospitals, and established doctor to doctor contacts for referral. With the advent of the NHS, it became necessary to create a progressive career structure for doctors who were to work within the state health care system, especially since it became likely that all or most of a medical career would be within it. Although in the period before the NHS, senior doctors usually had assistants in a quasi post-qualification apprenticeship system, the career structure in the newly established NHS concentrated on junior doctors who would be subject to the authority of more senior doctors. The chain therefore progressed from house officer (HO), to senior house officer (SHO), to registrar, senior registrar (all designated as junior doctors) to consultant. The implementation of this system was a further incentive, on top of allowing part-time private practice which had been conceded at its inception, to encourage senior consultants to enter and support the new NHS. The clinical firm, therefore, comprised a practical, small group of doctors working as a team in the same specialty and hospital. Typically, it would consist of one or two consultants and a variable constellation of junior doctors, depending, for example, on whether the hospital was a teaching hospital or not.

The influence of the medical career structure

Officially, newly qualified doctors must complete two periods of six months in pre-registration HO posts in recognised hospital specialties, frequently but not exclusively in general medicine or general surgery. Following completion of these posts to the satisfaction of the consultants for whom the HO has been working, full registration of the doctor with the General Medical Council may take place. Broadly speaking, doctors' career paths bifurcate at this point. One group undertakes vocational training for general practice and the other sets out on the route towards becoming a hospital consultant.

Vocational training for general practice involves three years experience, at least twelve months of which are in approved (by the Royal Colleges) hospital posts (usually at SHO level) in defined specialties and twelve months as a trainee general practitioner. Those taking the hospital specialty path are required firstly to undergo three years of General Professional Training (GPT) in approved hospital SHO or registrar posts. The intention of this GPT period is for the young doctor to obtain a broad experience in medicine. However, there is intense competition in the popular specialties since entry to the necessary higher professional examinations run by the Royal Colleges often requires particular kinds of hospital experience during the GPT period. For example, those wishing to become consultants in general medicine must obtain the Membership of the Royal College of Physicians (MRCP) examination which requires that not less than twelve months should be spent in posts involving the care of emergency medical patients, usually during the GPT period (Royal College of Physicians of London, 1988). Accreditation in a specialty depends on further experience of about four years in Higher Medical Training (HMT). Although accreditation is not mandatory for appointment to the consultant grade, it is widely accepted in the profession as an eligibility criterion. These posts are mainly at senior registrar grade and are approved by the Joint Committee on Higher Medical Training (JCHMT), a body mainly composed of representatives of the Royal Colleges, University departments and specialty associations (Joint Committee on Higher Medical Training, 1991). Two main points emerge from the requirements of training in medicine after qualification. Firstly, although there is some flexibility, most career pathways for doctors include prescribed experience of some kind and, therefore, career goals and commitments are usually set at an early stage. Secondly, training programmes suggested by the JCHMT in certain specialties, for example general medicine, recommend that experience in hospital administration is an important component of training and attendance at a management course is encouraged. There are, however, no data to confirm or otherwise the extent to which such recommendations are met.

For the most part, the relationship between consultants and junior doctors is based on authority conferred by specialist skills and an educational relationship whereby knowledge, skills and attitudes in medicine are transferred from senior to junior. In practice, however, the relationship also appears to be strongly influenced by a managerial, hierarchical authority. This is stimulated by the short-term nature of junior doctor appointments and, therefore, the continual need for advancement from one appointment to the next. Such progress is necessary because training programmes, including those for general practice, as noted above are largely specialty based. Further, there are few substantive job opportunities in medicine until a doctor reaches consultant level in the hospital-based specialties or 'principal' status in general practice. This means that steps sideways off the career ladder in one specialty and onto a rung at a similar level on the career ladder in another are often difficult to take. A change of interest, failure to advance or disillusionment in one specialty often requires a restart, frequently near the bottom rung of the training ladder of another.

These specialty-based training structures are reinforced by the requirements for fulfilment of the criteria of the Committees of Medical Training. These require, for example, that a specified period of time has been spent in a particular specialty in a particular grade. As medicine becomes increasingly specialised – there are some 80 recognised sub-specialties – the narrowness of the career path for an aspiring junior doctor within a particular specialty is apparent. The junior is highly dependent, therefore, on a good report and reference from the consultant of the clinical firm of his current post. It is worth noting in this context that trainees in the specialty of public health medicine, for whom the short course in organisation and management described later in this chapter was designed, are also subject to the regulations of GPT and HMT noted earlier. In contrast, however, it is somewhat atypical in that the specialty attracts and accommodates entrants at a more mature career stage than many others. That is to say, there is a wide variation in the prior clinical experience of entrants to the specialty of public health medicine. For instance, some will opt for a career in the specialty at an early stage during the period of GPT whereas others reach senior positions in other fields of medical practice before switching into public health medicine training. The specialty of public health medicine is concerned with the assessment of the need for and planning (or purchasing) of clinical and preventive services in order to create the best health for the population of a health authority. It is not perhaps surprising, therefore, that the specialty has recognised its particular need for organisational analysis, using both technical and behavioural skills as described in the following section, in order to achieve an appropriate outcome in working with others.

A framework for the analysis of Health Care organisations

The two broad functions of an organisation, in the course of pursuing organisational objectives, are the complementary processes of maintaining and controlling the organisation whilst enacting necessary change. Each of these tasks fulfils the conventional definition of management, that is, getting things done through people. Two distinct but interdependent qualities are required for getting things done, namely technical knowledge and skills on the one hand and behavioural or people skills on the other. Diagram 1.1, below, sets out some of the skills that fall under these headings. As noted earlier, relatively little has been written concerning the behavioural aspects of doctors as managers yet health services literature is replete with management as a technical activity in health care. In many ways, the current stage of development in management training for doctors mirrors the post-war professional training of doctors. The science

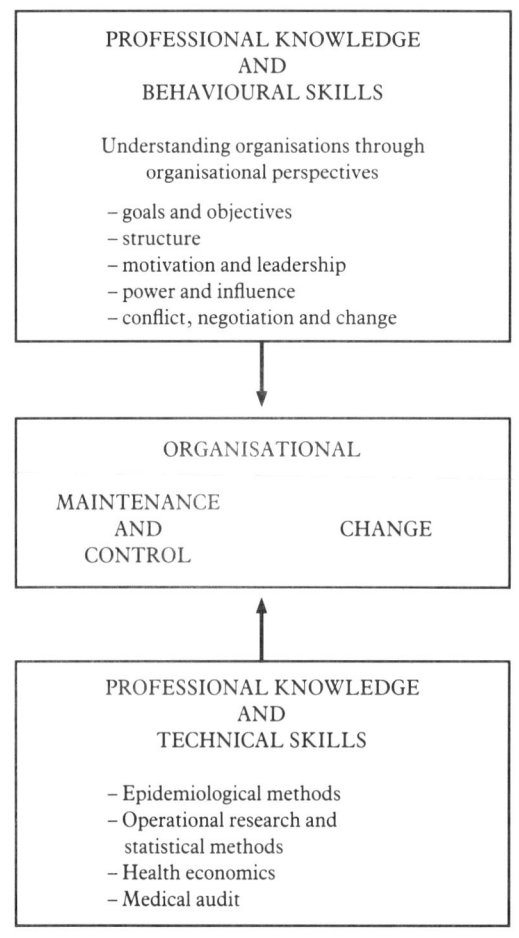

Diagram 1.1 An evaluative framework for Health Services management

of medicine dominated the curriculum and only relatively recently have behavioural issues such as the sociological aspects of medicine, communication with patients and the care of the dying found their way onto the agenda (General Medical Council, 1980).

A simple illustration from a 1984 seminar, though not directly involving doctors as managers, emphasises the need for a behavioural approach. A group of twelve unit (hospital) administrators, who were preparing to become unit general managers following the Griffiths proposals and who might have been expected to have been even more aware than doctors of behavioural issues in management, were given two minutes to prepare for the arrival of a foreign visitor, interested in NHS matters. Their brief was to write down the key words that they associated with the process of NHS planning at that time. The terms which predominated were 'needs', 'priorities', 'guidelines', 'information', 'resources', and 'evaluation'. The words used were in line with the expectations of the seminar leaders, ie terms associated with the language of the rational comprehensive planning model. The seminar leaders were then able to demonstrate to the participants how infrequently key words associated with a behavioural approach had been used eg 'persuasion', 'collaboration' and 'motivation' (Stuart Haywood, personal communication). In other words, these managers appeared to see their jobs primarily in terms of the technical half of evaluative skills summarised in Diagram 1.1, and saw little or no place for the role of behavioural factors. While this book concentrates on the other half of the diagram and focuses on behavioural aspects of health care organisations, many of the issues it deals with can only be understood in the wider context of the other, 'technical' elements in health care evaluation which, for the present at least, dominate the scene and many people's perception of what evaluation means. We therefore summarise, briefly, in turn the role of epidemiology, operational research and statistical methods, health economics and medical audit, outlining the nature of the principal technical mechanisms of management in the health service.

Diagram 1.1 sets out the themes relevant to a particular organisation (or department – which for the purposes of analysis here will be regarded as an organisation) that will be considered. It should be noted that for the purposes of explanation, it is necessary to pluck the theoretical element out of the framework and describe it as a rather circumscribed entity. However, although each element (for example, leadership) is distinguishable in its own right and has characteristics of its own, the characteristics of the organisation as a whole will depend, not only on leadership but on the interrelationship of all the elements (power, influence, epidemiological insights and so on) within the organisation. Moreover, the overall attributes of an organisation depend also on the wider environment in which the organisation exists.

In short, the way in which an organisation works as a whole is derived from more than the sum of its parts or elements. One purpose of the Case Studies, to be described later, is to indicate the effects of these internal and external interrelationships. This approach is well known in the field of individual psychology, particularly that of Gestalt psychology, in which purely psychological explanations of personality are found to be inadequate and socio-cultural forces also have to be taken into account. That is to say, personality is fluid or dynamic in that it is influenced by a person's environment.

Professional knowledge and technical skills

Epidemiological methods

Traditionally, epidemiological methods were directed at exploring the natural history and cause of disease. More recently, however, epidemiology has been increasingly involved in studies of the distribution and frequency of disease for the purposes of planning health services. In the recently changed NHS, planning which used to involve cooperation between managers and professionals, has been replaced by a quasi-market mechanism in which health authorities, responsible for the health of a defined resident population, assess its health care needs. The health authority then purchases health care from provider hospitals or services (Secretaries of State for Health, Wales, Northern Ireland and Scotland, 1989).

The assessment of health care needs has been interpreted largely as an epidemiological process in which the various methods of the discipline are used to measure the frequency and severity of diseases or conditions in the health authority's population. An added condition in the definition of a health care need is that an effective form of health care exists (though is not necessarily currently provided) for the prevention or treatment of the condition. Epidemiology, through the use of techniques such as randomised controlled trials, is again the discipline which is predominantly involved in the measurement of effectiveness; that is the improvement of the course of the disease or condition for the better.

Operational Research (OR) and statistical methods

It could be argued that epidemiological studies represent an examination of what is measurable in objective terms of current health needs and the effectiveness of health services and treatments. In the field of health services management, in particular, operational research involves the use of a set of mathematical and statistical techniques to examine and predict what will happen in a process of change. Mathematical models and computer simulation techniques allow OR scientists to explore the different outcomes likely given a range of possible resource inputs (often constrained), and differing ways of using such inputs. For example, commonly explored problems have included appointment systems in hospitals and general practice and improving the use of hospital beds (Flagle, 1962).

Health economics

As the proportion of GNP taken up by health care has increased in developed countries, regardless of whether in the public or private sector, nations have been seeking ways of curtailing health expenditure. Increasingly, therefore, health economics has been used as a rational approach to this dilemma by the investigation of ways of utilising potentially available health care resources to produce maximum health benefits. The development of health economics as a discipline has been possible because of the concurrent advances in epidemiology in the measurement of the effectiveness and health benefits of health care. An economic analysis can only be as good as the medical or epidemiological results on which the economics is superimposed. In brief, health economics' techniques involve cost-effectiveness and cost-utility studies (finding the least costly way of achieving desirable health outcomes, relative values being placed on the outcomes in the latter), and cost-benefit analysis (the costs and beneficial consequences of different programmes aimed at improving health are compared in money terms) (Drummond et al, 1987).

Medical audit

The fundamental objective of medical audit is to improve the quality of health care that doctors and other professionals provide for patients. The key features of audit are that it should be structured, systematic and quantifiable (Department of Health, 1990). Most medical audit, in a similar manner to epidemiological studies, depends on quantifiable data provided by routine or *ad hoc* information systems. What is uncertain is the way in which medical audit brings about changes in medical practice, that is to say, how are the quantitative features of the audit investigation converted into the necessary behavioural changes.

We would argue that any comprehensive strategy for the evaluation of health care systems must remain fatally flawed while the technical approaches reviewed here remain uncomplemented by a related evaluation of the behavioural aspects of the organisations concerned. It is to those aspects that we now turn.

Understanding organisations

In this part of the Introduction, in order to provide a context for the individual accounts of doctors in action as managers which are presented in this book and, in particular, to explain the theoretical background to their work, we outline the organisation and management section of the MSc course for which the contributions were orginally written. After a brief summary of the structure of the course, we provide a synoptic introduction to the main theoretical concepts considered in the course. This is intended to give the non-specialist in organisational behaviour some idea of the main tools of analysis employed by the students in their case studies. It can also be used as a source of further reading for those who want to explore the subject further.

The organisation and management course

Both the MSc in Public Health Medicine and the professional qualification of Membership of the Faculty of Public Health Medicine (MFPHM) for which the contributors were studying include a requirement that students should be familiar with central concepts in the organisation and management literature and show an ability to apply them to practical issues in the field of public health medicine. The organisation and management course is designed both to help students meet these requirements and to provide a solid introduction to the field which those who are so inclined can also use as a foundation for further exploration later on. The course emphasises for all students, however, the importance of developing the application of the concepts they have studied in the field. To this end it includes a small project focusing on the analysis of some aspect either of the organisation in which they are currently working, or some other health organisation in which they have previously worked.

The structure of the course

The course is divided into five sections:
- An overview of the development of organisation theory and related perspectives on the nature and role of management
- A review of major theoretical perspectives and ways in which they can be applied in organisational analysis

- The projects in which students apply theoretical perspectives to a practical organisational setting known to them
- The presentation of the projects to the group and learning from this
- A review of cross-cutting themes identified in the previous stages of the course such as power, professionalism, and the management of change

The emphasis in this short course is placed firmly on developing an analytical approach to organisations rather than on attempting to introduce a range of specific managerial skills. The course is necessarily introductory in nature and students are not expected to acquire a sophisticated understanding of the field in the limited time available. Nevertheless, it provides a sufficient foundation on which to build a systematic view of behaviour in organisations and, as the Case Studies suggest, can be put to practical use in enhancing students' understanding of the organisations in which they work.

The theoretical underpinning of the course

Organisational theory, like the wider field of social theory of which it is part, is an area of contested explanations (see, eg, Reed, 1985; Reed and Hughes, 1993). It is not our intention here to explore and detail these, but it is relevant to indicate where the approach taken in the course lies in relation to the wider theoretical context. In a useful overview of the subject, Burrell and Morgan (1979), draw a distinction between theories of society based on the view of the centrality of order, stability and integration, and those which stress the importance of conflict, coercion and change. The former they describe as the sociology of regulation and the latter as the sociology of radical change.

Most contemporary organisational theory can be seen as falling within the sociology of regulation. This is, perhaps, only to be expected, given that most industrial sociologists, psychologists, industrial relations specialists and the like are employed directly or indirectly by those with interests in maintaining the existing social structure. There is much less current work, particularly in terms of empirical studies, based on more radical views which emphasise differences of interest and interpretation of what organisations are and do in contemporary society, and of how this wider society itself may be understood. The theoretical perspective taken in the course provided for the MSc in Public Health Medicine is weighted towards the perspective of regulatory sociology, although it gives due emphasis to the importance of recognising the effect of the different interpretations that different actors place on what some people might call the 'same' situation, and the significance of change and conflict in understanding any organisational context. This starting point for the course, it may be added, is not derived from the view that the positivist approach (believing in an absolute knowledge) that is often associated with it is correct, and that there is a single reality 'out there', regardless of our personal perceptions. Rather, it stems from the position that reality is socially constructed and that at any one time particular definitions of it, usually those supported by the most established and powerful groups in a society, have the upper hand. These definitions are central to an understanding of what those in control of most organisations are trying to do and how they are setting about doing it.

For this reason the first and larger part of the course examines concepts which help to explain how organisations are seen and structured by those in control of them, perspectives which are predominantly positivist in orientation. However, the second part of the course recognises the importance of exploring the perceptions, experience and behaviour of all the actors in any organisational setting, and not just those of their controllers. In this way, what some sociologists have called an 'action perspective' is introduced, stressing that people are not simply passive recipients of the social forces to which they are subject, but act back on and influence their own environments in their turn. So it becomes important to understand these processes too, to explore differences of interest, and to analyse outcomes in conflict and negotiation.

Within this framework, the theoretical core of the course falls into a logical sequence of six main sections. These can also be used by the students as steps in the analysis of their own organisations and methods of undertaking such analyses are discussed with them at the end of each section. For the purpose of the course the unit of analysis may be a discrete, bounded organisation such as a general practice, or a part (sub-system) of a much larger organisation such as a hospital ward or an operating theatre. Carefully applied, most of the concepts considered can be used equally well at either level.

1. Organisational variety

Early theories tended to assume a unitary view of organisations. As the American engineer F.W. Taylor, the 'father' of Scientific Management put it, there must be 'one best way' to undertake any activity and the job of managers was to identify it and structure matters accordingly (Taylor, 1947). Much the same message can be found in the influential work of Max Weber who saw bureaucracy as the dominant type of organisation in modern society and who, although he was well aware of its limitations and dangers, believed there was no viable alternative for large scale enterprises and dismissed attempts to create them as mere 'dilettantism' (Weber, 1947 p.337). However, more recent students have noted that the successful implementation of different tasks and different technologies seems to require substantial differences in organisational structure and management, including, for instance, the extent to which it is advantageous for organisations to be flexible and organic or fixed and mechanistic (see, eg, Kast and Rosenzweig, 1985). This 'contingency approach' to organisations is examined in the course with a particular focus on the work of Henry Mintzberg. Mintzberg has identified a number of key organisational configurations which provides a useful typology within which students can locate their own organisations (Mintzberg, 1979 and 1989) and gain some overall understanding of their structure and dynamics before grappling in more detail with the subject. The value of this approach in establishing an understanding of the nature of organisational variety justifies a rather fuller summary of the concepts involved than is devoted to other elements in the course.

Mintzberg prefers the term 'configuration' to contingency in his approach, identifying as he does the organised whole of his different types. The configurations are related to different patterns of key elements and coordinating mechanisms in organisations. The key elements are the *operating core*, carrying out the productive activity of the organisation; the *strategic apex* or top management; the *middle line* between the operating core and the strategic apex; the *technostructure* made up of specialist advisers and analysts; the *support staff*; and the *ideology or culture* of the organisation. The key coordinating mechanisms through which the different parts of an organisation are brought together into a functioning whole are mutual adjustment, direct supervision, standardisation of work processes, standardisation of outputs, standardisation of skills and knowledge, and standardisation of norms.

The classification of the prime coordinating mechanisms and key parts of an organisation, and relating these to the type of centralisation or decentralisation which predominates in an organisation, suggests the identification of seven main types of configuration: entrepreneurial, machine, professional, innovative, missionary, diversified, and political. For introductory purposes we can concentrate on the first five of these types since the diversified organisation is usually a sub-type of the machine organisation and the political organisation refers mainly to temporary phases in other configurations when intense political activity swamps normal functioning. It should be emphasised, however, that while this system of classification seems to work well in capturing the distinctive characteristics of most organisations, like all such schemes that attempt to distill the essence of highly complex human institutions, it is necessarily a simplification of reality. Organisations tend to be one or other of the configurations, and some are obviously hybrids or combinations of different configurations (Mintzberg, 1989 pp 265–70). The five main configurations are:

The entrepreneurial organisation is essentially a personal organisation. The key part of its structure is the top leadership, often a single individual.

All power and coordination focus at this point. Many large, complex organisations begin life as small-scale entrepreneurial organisations before they evolve into machine or professional bureaucracies. In the health field entrepreneurial organisations are often found in the private sector in specialist clinics, nursing homes, health farms and so on. But elements of the entrepreneurial approach can often also be identified within the public sector in general practice (see, for instance, Case Studies 9 and 10) and within other kinds of organisation as, for example, where a medical 'firm' in a hospital, developing new treatments, seeks to promote its work far beyond the normal catchment area of the institution.

The machine organisation is typically concerned with highly routinised activities and standardised products. The technostructure is the key part of the organisation since it is this section which designs the standardised work procedures on which all operations are based. Coordination is achieved primarily through the standardisation of technology. This configuration fits quite closely with Max Weber's classical definition of the bureaucratic organisation (Weber, 1947) which described its basis in legal-rational authority, specialised, highly sub-divided work tasks, hierarchy, rules, the appointment and promotion of staff on the basis of qualifications or tested competence, and so on. Obvious examples of the machine organisation are the mass production factory, the army and the government department. In health organisations, large hospitals usually have strongly developed machine characteristics in their administrative and nursing hierarchies. Case Studies 4 and 5, in particular, describe situations in which machine features of the hospital were key factors.

The professional organisation tends to emerge wherever the operating work of an enterprise 'is dominated by skilled workers who use procedures that are difficult to learn yet are well defined.' (Mintzberg, 1989, p.181). The professional organisation is like the machine organisation in that the skills of staff are standardised, but it differs crucially from it in that the standards are established outside the organisation, in the training of the professionals, and that the day-to-day work of the professionals requires the exercise of considerable discretion (Ackroyd, Hughes & Soothill, 1989). Thus the key part of the professional organisation is its front-line staff and the main coordinating mechanism is the standardised nature of their special skills. The university, the law firm, and the architectural practice are all typical professional organisations.

Health organisations tend to conform to the professional configuration where the professionals dominate as, potentially, in general practice and in doctor controlled hospitals. Large public hospitals, which provide the setting for most of the Case Studies in this book, are likely to combine both machine or bureaucratic elements (in the administrative hierarchy) and professional and entrepreneurial elements (in the medical firms), together with the mixed machine-professional element of the nursing hierarchy (Case Studies 1,2,4–7).

The innovative organisation occurs where the main business of an enterprise is change and creativity. Typically, such organisations, which include activities as diverse as those of fashion houses, advertising agencies, consultancy firms, and guerrilla bands operating behind enemy lines have loose, adaptable structures; their staff work in project or task teams rather than established hierarchies, and mutual adjustment is their main coordinating mechanism. Innovative organisations are not typical of health services which are primarily concerned with the provision of standard, predictable outputs. However, research and development sections of health organisations which are dominated by professional or machine characteristics, may exhibit much in common with innovative enterprises. Similarly, a general practice can go through phases when a strong innovative element is added to what is otherwise properly defined as a professional organisation, as two of the case studies reported in this book illustrate (Case Studies 9 and 10).

The missionary organisation emerges where the main driving force is the shared beliefs of its members. Any kind of crusading organisation, not only the obvious example of religious missions, can fall into this category. Voluntary bodies promoting a particular cause, for example saving the environment, protecting children or animals, may have this character. The standardisation of norms provides the main coordinating mechanism in such organisations and their key element is their particular ideology. Missionary organisations are unlikely to be encountered in the public health service but voluntary organisations representing the interests of various categories of patients such as those suffering from a particular disease or disability can often have missionary characteristics, especially early in their life-cycles when they are new and small.

2. Control

When it has been successfully established what type of configuration best describes an organisation, the student is well placed to move on to the analysis of the location of power and authority as the next step to gaining an understanding of organisational goals, structure and management. As a preliminary in this process it is important to explore the concepts of power and authority and to show that they are not necessarily synonymous: people can be vested with the authority to run an organisation or part of it but for various reasons not command the power that they need to actually get things done. Or they may have no formal authority in an organisation and yet acquire real power by other means to influence or even control decisions.

Beyond a person's official position, other sources of power which have been identified by students of organisations include expertise, reward –

control over valued resources, coercion, and personal qualities (sometimes called referent power) (French and Raven, 1970). From this standpoint it becomes clear that it can often be possible for people at lower levels in an organisation to wield considerable power and influence. A classic study of factors which could enhance the power of 'lower participants' in organisations drew attention to the importance of access to information, length of service, expertise, irreplaceability, willingness to inject effort, personal attractiveness, and the centrality of location of the individual's job (Mechanic, 1962). Even the apparently most powerless who have few or none of these specific advantages, we should add, have the very real potential negative power of being able to withold their wholehearted consent from the performance of their roles.

How power of all kinds is distributed in an organisation is discussed at a later stage in the course when the interaction of different interest groups is considered. However, in attempting to define the locus of the effective controlling group it is important to recognise that in all but the smallest organisations, the need to coordinate the different component parts means that in practice power is usually wielded by a group of leaders. This is often most appropriately understood as a coalition rather than a command hierarchy. Given that there may be other coalitions within the organisation, this directing group has come to be described by some students as the dominant coalition (Child, 1972; Kotter, 1978).

3. Goals and their implementation

The identification of the controller or controllers in an organisation facilitates the isolation of the goals that are being pursued by those with the power to direct it. At this stage a systems perspective is introduced to help identify what the controllers see as their main tasks and how they conceptualise the process of structuring and running the organisation to achieve them. The case for using a systems approach in this exercise is not based on a judgement of the value of the perspective in describing organisational behaviour, but on the assumption that it is likely to represent quite effectively the way in which most controllers actually perceive their situation and how they need to act. The definition of tasks, the logical identification of steps to be taken to complete the tasks based on an analysis of the technical processes required, and the structuring of organisations round those processes draw on the well-established example of scientific management. Systems thinking, with its emphasis on the interrelation of different systems with each other and on the role of subsystems within systems, builds on this approach by providing what many managers regard as a helpful framework for conceptualising the wider environment of an organisation (seeing it as an 'open' system) and its impact on its internal operation.

There are numerous ways of conceptualising organisations as systems (see, eg, Checkland, 1981). The course focuses on the widely used socio-technical systems approach developed by researchers at the Tavistock Institute which goes beyond some more process-orientated models in the emphasis it gives to the social dimensions of the organisation of the enterprise (Trist and Bamforth, 1951; Rice, 1960; Miller and Rice, 1967). Drawing on a biological perspective which sees living organisms as systems seeking homeostasis through an exchange with their environment, organisations are defined as open systems similarly earning their survival and development through a process of inputs, conversion, and outputs which are exchanged for further inputs. A key distinction which can be derived from this approach is that between the task or tasks that must be fulfilled to ensure the survival of the organisation (the primary task or tasks) and other activities pursued by the organisation (which can be defined as secondary tasks or 'mission' tasks).

The first step in the analysis of any organisation is to identify the primary task or tasks. From this starting point the socio-technical systems analyst can set out to establish the three key subsystems which all organisations require: the productive system, the maintenance system, and the regulatory system. The productive system is concerned with the conversion of inputs into outputs defined by the primary task, as for example, turning raw materials into a finished product in a factory or treating patients requiring treatment in a hospital. The maintenance system provides the essential support services to the productive system such as the supply of tools, heating, lighting, and the recruitment of personnel. The regulatory system focuses on the boundaries of the systems and subsystems of the productive and maintenance systems, assessing their performance and feeding back information to other parts of the organisation to trigger any adjustments required to ensure the fulfilment of the primary task. A key part of systems analysis is the identification of appropriate boundaries between systems and subsystems. Where organisations are pursuing secondary or mission tasks as well as primary or survival tasks, the same methods of analysis can be applied to these and to their relation to the primary task or tasks. The student must also seek to understand how organisations in addition to their work-related systems, have social and psychological properties. Where the work organisation fails to meet important needs related to these properties their performance is likely to be adversely affected. Looking specifically at the basic unit of the front-line team, for example, this may well come to acquire meaning and importance for its members beyond its formal task, based on shared experience and feelings. The workings of such 'sentient groups' as the Tavistock researchers called them, are ignored at management's peril (Miller and Rice, 1967).

Several of the Case Studies contained in this book draw on this approach to systems analysis. They illustrate the applicability of the method not only to whole organisations, as in the case of the general practices described in Case Studies 8, 9 and 10 but also to subsystems of larger systems, even when the workings of the larger system may be obscure to the analyst, as in the examples of hospital ward organisation in Case Studies 1, 4, and 5.

4. Gaining compliance

The first modern writers on organisation appeared to believe that once an appropriate system of production had been established gaining the compliance of the workforce who would run it was relatively simple. The most adequate motivation was likely to require a scheme of rewards and punishments, relating compliance and output to pay and security. This view of motivation was clearly indicated, for example, in the scientific management methods of F.W. Taylor, referred to above (p. 20). He first detailed what he saw as the system of production required by the logic of the technical processes involved, and then established measures of individual performance which were linked directly to bonuses for good performance, and loss of pay and the threat of the sack for poor performance (Taylor, 1947). The possibility of appealing to other motives such as personal development, the intrinsic interest of the job, or relationships with fellow workers does not seem to have occurred to him. However, as organisations have become more complex, workforces more educated, skilled and better organised in unions and professional associations, this concentration on simple, extrinsic motives for working, has been increasingly challenged and more sophisticated models of motivation have been developed. The course examines, in particular, two phases in this process, the emergence of the human relations school, and subsequent work based on 'complex' man.

The human relations school, whose origins can be traced back to the famous Hawthorne studies of Elton Mayo and his colleagues in the 1920s and 1930s, is based on the view that people bring far more needs to work than simply the need to make a living (Mayo, 1933; Roethlisberger and Dickson, 1939). Mayo's work convinced him that in modern, anomic society, workers wanted a workplace where they could realise their need for a sense of belonging and personal significance. Subsequent researchers, drawing on the work of humanistic psychologists such as Abram Maslow, Eric Fromm and Carl Rogers, have broadened the concept of workers' needs still further and argue for the recognition of the potential for personal development and self-actualisation in the way that all work is organised (eg Maslow, 1954; 1965; Fromm, 1956; Rogers, 1972).

Douglas McGregor's well-known *Theory X* and *Theory Y* encapsulates the contrasting position of the scientific management and human relations approaches to motivation (McGregor, 1960). *Theory X* is based on the economic man model of motivation. It argues that most people do not like working and are only motivated to work by extrinsic rewards and punishments. For the same reason, when they are at work they cannot be trusted to get on with their jobs under their own steam but have to be closely supervised and controlled. Indeed, most people prefer things to be organised in this way and shun taking on responsibilities. In contrast, *Theory Y* posits that the desire to work, in the sense of making and creating things, is as natural to human beings as the desire to rest and to play. If people come to react negatively in the work place it is because of their long experience of being denied opportunities for significant and satisfying roles there. The challenge for managers of modern organisations, it follows, is to restructure them so that they can offer their members every opportunity to develop and to realise their higher level needs. In this way a positive synergy will be produced in which the individual and the organisation contribute to the mutual satisfaction of their needs.

Theory Y had profound implications for the organisation of work including the need to move away from technological determinism in the structuring of jobs towards creating work tasks that could be personally fulfilling and the replacement of directive, authoritarian styles of management by more participative, or democratic styles. Rensis Likert's work has explored the implementation of such alternatives. He starts from a typology of four key styles of management which he believes can be identified in contemporary organisations: (1) exploitive authoritative, (2) benevolent authoritative, (3) consultative, and (4) participative. He shows how each style is associated with different patterns of organisational structure and process and that styles 3 and 4 appear to be superior both from the point of view of meeting the needs of the organisation and of its members. In an examination of these last two styles of management he shows how they can be fostered through the use of decentralised, semi-autonomous groups, with overlapping membership linking them into a coherent whole (Likert, 1967).

These and other human relations or neo-human relations approaches to motivation are readily grasped and appeal to many students of organisations as being far more compatible with the values of a would-be democratic society than those of the scientific management school. They have in their turn, nevertheless, come under the close scrutiny of researchers and have been criticised by some for over simplification (eg Silverman, 1970; Butler, 1986; Maccoby 1988). In particular, it has been argued that even if all human beings have the potential for personal development and self-realisation, they may not wish or be able to pursue it, or they may deliberately choose to do so in their non-work lives while approaching the choice of work instrumentally, in ways which maximise their opportunities to follow such a strategy (eg Goldthorpe and Lockwood et al, 1968). These scholars believe that in any particular organisational context it is more useful to start with a complex model of people's motivation, not assuming in advance that it will be intelligible in terms of a particular hierarchy of needs, but rather that it should be understood in terms of different hierarchies and different priorities at different times or in terms of different character types (eg Schein, 1980; Maccoby, 1988). This model, it will be apparent, also sits more comfortably with the contingency approach to organisations which is introduced at the beginning of the course. Different types of organisation, other things being equal, can be expected to be more compatible with different motivational strategies and to attract (where there is choice) people with different expectations and needs. Thus professional organisations with their emphasis on collegiality, and innovative organisations with their reliance on self-starting teams, are more likely to need members with an internalised commitment to their work and consultative or participative leadership while machine organisations may tend to authoritative styles and emphasise instrumental motivation.

By this stage in the course the students have been introduced to a set of conceptual tools which they can use to construct a picture of an organisation from the perspective of those seeking to control and manage it. However, as the discussion of the issue of motivation has made clear, the controllers do not hold all the cards in the organisational game. To try to understand the organisation in its totality it is essential to gain a clear view of how the other participants see and experience their membership, and how this in turn influences their behaviour.

5. The view from below
The sociological perspective which lends itself most readily to this task is the action frame of reference. This starts from the assumption that while human beings are shaped and influenced by the social structures and processes of the world in which they live, they also in their turn act in ways which can change those forces. It begins, therefore, with an assessment of the ways in which different actors are motivated, the nature of their commitment to their roles, their perceptions of the current situation, the actions they may be taking to try to change the situation and their resulting interaction with each other and the controllers. In what is necessarily a simplifying process, some way is needed to condense the complexities of motivation and definitions of the situation. For example, involvement of people can be defined as moral (commitment to the goals and norms of the organisation), calculative or instrumental (interest in extrinsic rewards received from working there), or alienative (associated with hostile relationships or involuntary membership of the organisation as for example a prisoner, or conscript) (Etzioni, 1961).

The action perspective encourages an examination of how these factors relate to change and conflict within organisations and implies that at any one time the prevailing arrangements for management are likely to represent, at least in part, a negotiated rather than an imposed order and that renegotiation and change are intrinsic characteristics of all human institutions (eg Silverman, 1970). This approach opens a new vista on organisations in which the behaviour of organisation members is always seen as potentially problematic and may often be, in the eyes of management, perceived as deviant or even subversive. The work of social scientists on the role of defensive and aggressive cliques (eg Dalton, 1959; Lupton, 1963; Pettigrew, 1973), on both formal and informal negotiations between groups within them (e.g. Gouldner, 1954; Strauss et al 1971; Neuhauser, 1988), and on the power and influence of lower level members of organisations (eg Mechanic, 1962; Kearns, 1976; Watson, 1982) provides many examples of the dynamics of such behaviour and its impact.

The end result is often one in which the emergent picture of the organisation and the social relationships through which it operates from day to day – the negotiated order as opposed to the imposed order – is very different from the formal picture presented by management in organisation charts and rule books. Yet it is only by achieving some kind of an understanding of this negotiated order that sense can be made of the achievements and shortcomings of an organisation, however these are defined.

6. Outcomes: order and flux

This sequence of analytical steps concludes by considering ways of evaluating the outcome of the processes examined in terms of the nature of the order or flux prevailing and their consequences for the objectives of the controlling individual or group.

Finally, the implications of the subject matter of the course for policy formulation and implementation within the health service context are discussed with particular reference to contemporary issues. Specifically, the approach adopted in the course is used to review organisational change. This is first addressed, following Lewin (1947), by examining the force-field approach which focuses on the countervailing forces resisting and promoting change in any particular situation. This is applied in the context of contingency theory which makes it possible to illustrate the significance of different organisational contexts in understanding the process of change. So, for example, the machine organisation with its entrenched bureaucratic structure is typically highly resistant to change while in entrepreneurial and innovative organisations change is likely to be an accepted part of the culture. These perspectives, combined with the other conceptual tools developed in the course, provide a framework for the critical evaluation of various strategies for managing change from the classic work on participation (eg Coch and French, 1948; Likert, 1967) to more recent eclectic approaches (eg Kotter and Schlesinger, 1979; Kanter, 1983, 1992; Carnall, 1990).

The concentrated nature of the course makes considerable demands on students' intellectual digestive systems but to judge both from their own evaluations and from the character and standard of the project work they produce on organisations, they are well able to cope with it. While most are new to the social sciences, apart from an introductory course on sociology, the fact that all have already worked in several different organisational settings and are experienced organisation-watchers doubtless helps equip them to make use of the strengths of organisational theory and at the same time alerts them to its limitations.

The ten case studies which follow offer evidence of their ability to apply their learning to good effect and in so doing to enhance our understanding of the micro world of doctors as managers.

PART II

The case studies

Introduction to the case studies

The ten case studies presented in the following pages were all written initially as projects for the organisation and management component of the MSc in Public Health Medicine course at Newcastle University and have subsequently been revised for inclusion in this book. Details of each of the organisations involved have been altered to ensure their anonymity. It should also be emphasised that the nature of such accounts by participant observers in the organisations concerned represent personal perceptions of the situations described and in this sense are necessarily subjective. On the other hand, the writers had the considerable advantage over more objective observers on the outside, of experiencing the day-to-day operation of their organisations at first hand.

The wide range of settings represented is illustrative of the varied backgrounds of the doctors who are ultimately drawn to a career in public health medicine. However, the grouping of the studies under the headings of *equilibrium, conflict* and *change* reflects organisational dynamics rather than the formal structures and purposes of the institutions concerned. Most organisations which survive for any significant period of time experience all these states.

Equilibrium

Introduction

The three case studies which provided examples of equilibrium illustrate how the relative stability observed by their authors can arise from the satisfaction of key needs of their more important actors. This equilibrium can produce apparently effective work units (as in Case Studies 1 and 2) but it may also be the product of more flawed systems where a particular individual acquires and wields disproportionate power, and apparently achieves control by coercion and manipulation, as in Case Study 3. Equilibrium, whether underpinned by consensus or coercion can, as Case Study 1 shows, lead an organisation's leaders to develop a false sense of security, to neglect the importance of exchange relationships with the wider system of which it is part, and so to put its survival in jeopardy.

Case Study 1: The negotiated order in an acute surgical unit

A House Officer

Editors' introduction
This Case Study describes the stable relationships established within an acute surgical unit and how they contributed to the smooth running of its work. The focus of the study is on the roles and relationships of four key members of the unit in maintaining this equilibrium: the two consultants heading the surgical team, their senior registrar and a sister. The writer makes clear the crucial differences between the manifest organisation – its formal structure and distribution of authority and responsibilities – and the latent organisation. This distinction is essential to an understanding of the factors which accounted for the stable relationships at the core of the unit, including the satisfaction of the interests of all the key actors, and the

central role of the staff nurse in building and maintaining a participative style of leadership in what was on the surface a highly authoritarian set-up. However, the very factors which contributed to this particular brand of stability within the unit made it peculiarly vulnerable to changes in the wider environment of the hospital.

The setting for the case study was the post-Griffiths Report era of the NHS when general managers had been charged with increasing the efficiency of the service (DHSS and Griffiths, 1983). As part of the drive for efficiency, greater attention was being paid to the measurement of the performance of hospitals and units. In common with several of the other case studies described in this book, general management failed to influence the style of working of the professionals in this surgical firm. To their detriment, however, the members of the firm, unlike surgical colleagues elsewhere in the hospital, had failed to detect the change in ethos within the organisation. In addition, the perception of the function and performance of the firm in the context of the wider environment of the hospital as a whole was neglected by the professionals involved. The end result was the closure of the unit.

Organisational perspectives: to help describe the formal nature of the organisation of the unit, the writer draws on the work of Weber on the characteristics of bureaucracies (Introduction, page 20). However, his success in penetrating behind the facade of the authoritative structure is based on an effective use of an action perspective (Introduction, pages 28–9) to delineate the actual roles of the key actors in the two wards and to explore the interactions between them which produced the stable negotiated order which prevailed in the unit.

The Case Study

Making sense of the organisational culture of any large enterprise is no easy task and is necessarily influenced by one's personal perceptions. The NHS is no exception. There exist a great variety of different styles of leadership and many different patterns of organisation, as would be expected in so large a 'business'. This case study deals with a small corner of the NHS which nonetheless combined several of these styles. As a prelude to this account, Charles Handy's description of the powerfully placed individual in a traditional organisation, but whose inclination is for a 'person culture' which exists to serve and assist key professionals, provides an insightful view of how consultants often perceive their position in the hospital:

'... He does what he has to, teaches when he must, in order to retain his position in the organisation. But essentially he regards the organisation as a place where he can build his own career, carry out his own interests, all of which may indirectly add interest to the organisation though that would not be the point in doing them. ... Individuals with this orientation are not easy to manage. There is little power that can be brought to bear on them. Being specialists, alternative employment is often easy to obtain, or they have protected themselves by tenure, so that resource power has no potency. Position power not backed up by resource power achieves nothing. Expert power they are unlikely to acknowledge. Coercive power is not usually available, only personal power is left and such individuals are not easily impressed by personality' (Handy, 1985 p.196).

At the inception of the NHS the peculiar autonomy of the consultant within the perceived bureaucratic structure of the whole was carefully established. It has been maintained in the guise of clinical freedom ever since, even though the 'clinical' justification for such independence has been substantially discredited (Hampton, 1983; Hoffenburg, 1987). The right to 'clinical freedom' has in recent times become a metaphor for the right to one's own little kingdom, but the days of such personal kingdoms may well be coming to an end.

Manifest organisational structure

The 'king' in the situation I describe here is *Consultant X*, a surgeon in a large hospital. He is placed at the head of the structure shown in Diagram 2.1 which represents the commonly held view of the medical role culture of such a unit as this. This is clearly a picture of a bureaucratic structure, which appears to fulfil the Weberian criteria well; positions and roles are defined, appointment is by acquisition of qualifications, areas of work are legitimated to the post, and so on (Weber, 1947, pp.329–341). The position of the second *Consultant, Y*, is somewhat anomalous in this picture, as, although he supposedly shared the top position with his colleague *X*, in practice he had abdicated the role of leader.

Relating to this hierarchy in a rather ill-defined way is the nursing hierarchy represented in Diagram 2.2. In many respects the rigidity of the nursing bureaucracy tends to be greater than that of the medical. There is no formal path of responsibility linking the nursing to the medical hierarchy, but as an operational rule the lower order of the medical pyramid tends to communicate with the upper levels of the nursing equivalent (Diagram 2.3).

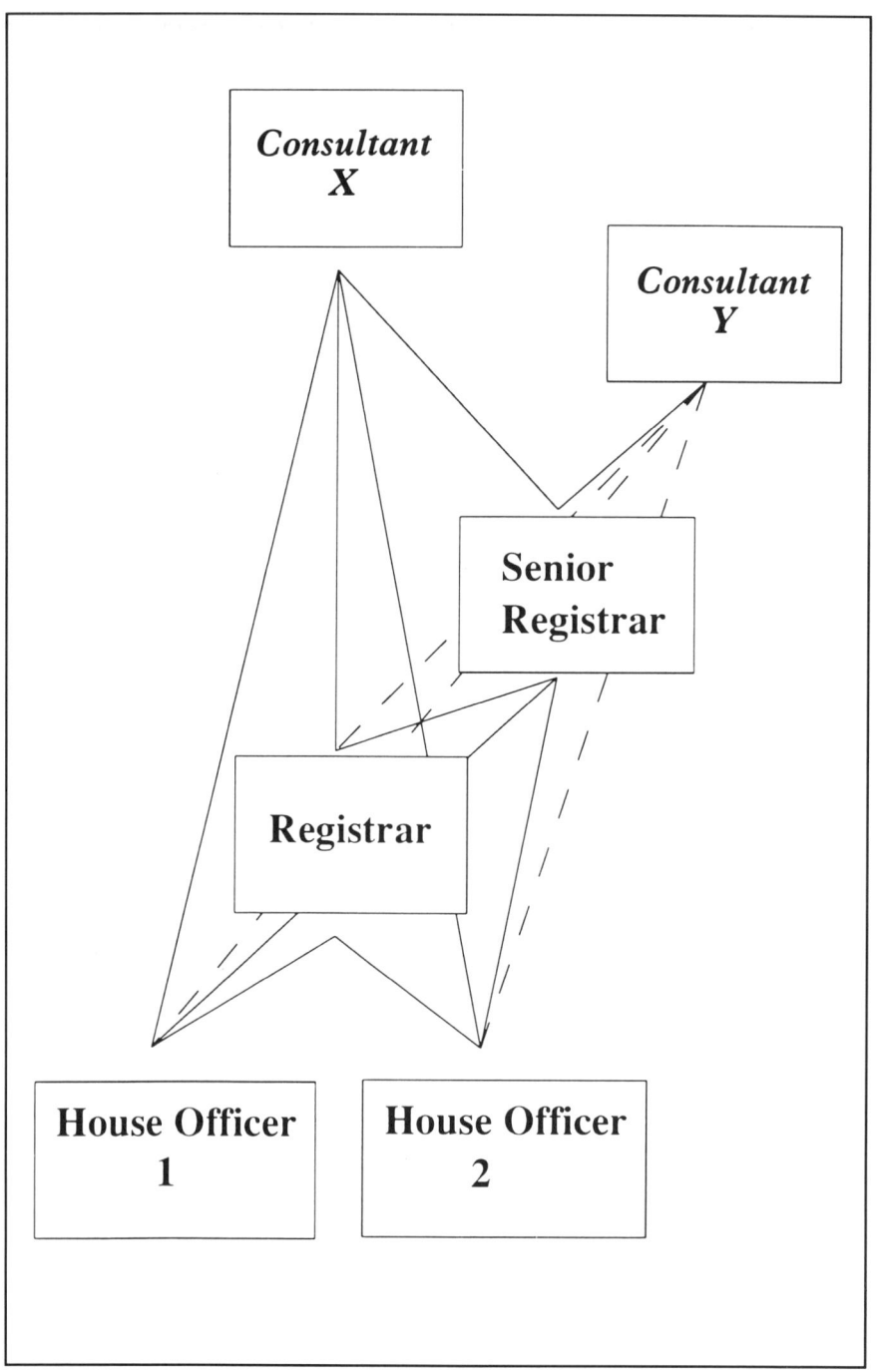

Diagram 2.1   The manifest organisational structure: Medical

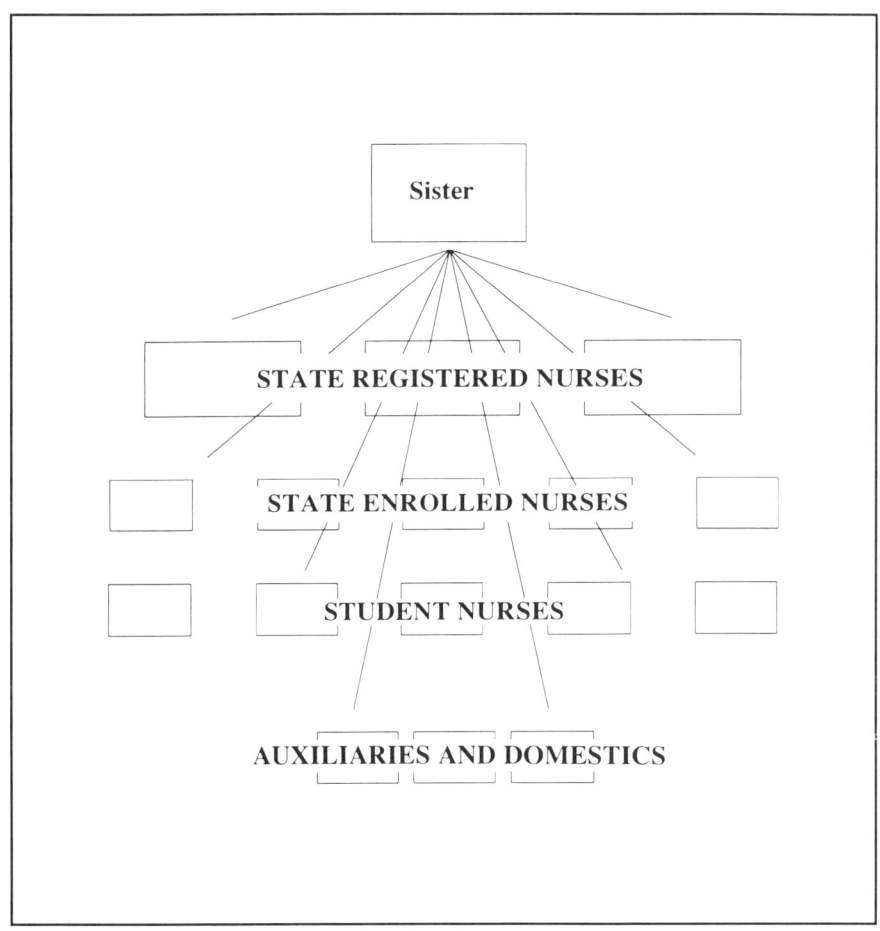

Diagram 2.2   The manifest organisational structure: Nursing

Within this unit there were, in fact, two separate nursing hierarchies attached to the two wards that comprised the unit, facing one another from opposite ends of a corridor and removed from the main body of the hospital. When I came to work on this unit my perception of the ward hierarchy was as described above, and the geographical separation of the wards from the rest of the hospital matched well the sensation of functional autonomy.

Medical actors
Consultant X, the central character, was an authoritarian consultant of the old school. In addition to his surgical consultancy he held a prestigious, mainly administrative, post in the medical school from which he practised belligerence toward the students. Other than this he had few teaching

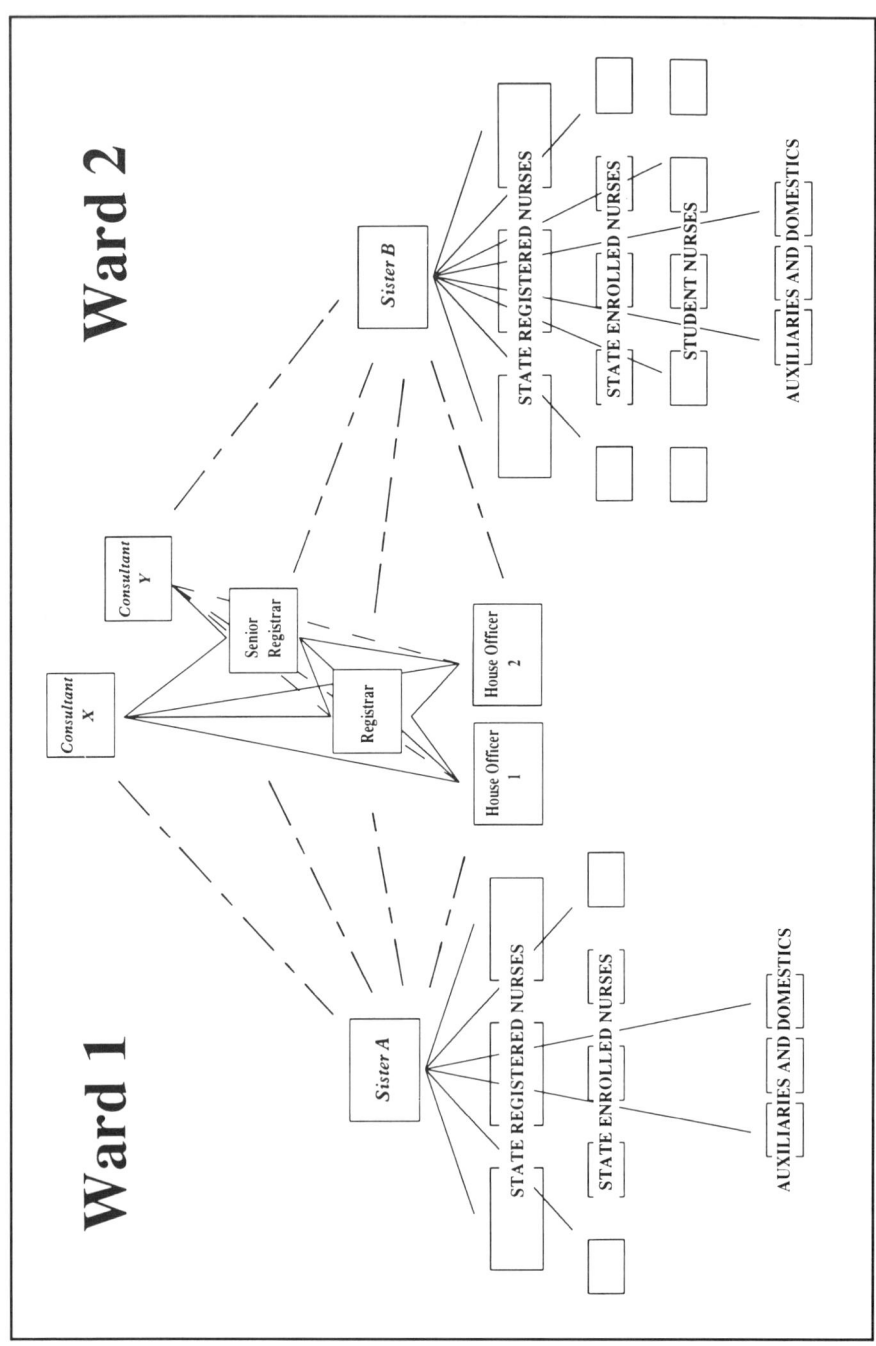

Diagram 2.3   The interrelationship of the manifest hierarchies
in the Acute Surgical Unit

commitments, and no active interest in research. To the casual observer there was no question that the two wards were X's surgical unit and that he was fully in control.

The working day for X followed a rigid routine, beginning at 7.30 am and finishing at 6.00 pm almost to the minute. He would spend the first hour of the day sitting in his office which was situated on the corridor leading to Ward 1. Very rarely did he have enough mail to keep him busy for this length of time, so he would often read a newspaper and smoke. His door was always open (in the literal sense) allowing him to see what time the juniors arrived for work. When late, it was not possible to sneak past without being seen – every time I thought I had managed to do so he would shout 'Good morning Dr . . .' down the passage to let me know that he had spotted me. It seemed to give him satisfaction to arrive on the ward and find a sleepless house officer (HO) at the desk before him – at such times he would even stop for a brief social chat. The junior staff were expected to commence a ward round at 8.15 am at which the business decisions were taken. In the meantime X would adjourn for coffee in the surgeon's room of the operating theatre and await the arrival of the first patient.

Patients were expected to arrive at theatre with notes, consent forms, all X-rays (relevant or not), and with the appropriate leg, hernial orifice, etc., signalled in blue felt pen. Failure to fulfil these conditions led to the house officer being summoned and humiliatingly dressed down in front of the patient. Virtually all of X's operations were done by himself, and even when the juniors were allowed to take over they were closely supervised. He was consistently rude to his medical staff during procedures but civil to the nurses and others. Once the list was completed, which was generally around lunchtime as X did not receive a large number of referrals, he would depart for the medical school for a few hours to deal with his administrative work there. This shortage of referrals arose partly because the professorial unit in the hospital insisted on keeping to itself all referrals addressed to the hospital, but not to any specific consultant, rather than distributing the cases among all of the surgeons on the site.

At 4.30 he returned to the ward and donned a white coat for his daily ward round at which he would see all of the patients, whether his or not. In contrast to the practice of his colleague Y, this was expected to be formal and every X-ray and lab report was to be seen by him. Understandably, this created a large amount of extra work in the afternoon as items were chased to different departments.

Consultant Y in stark contrast to his colleague X, was a clubbable and easy-going man whose hands-off approach to his NHS work allowed the senior registrar (SR) to function practically as a locum consultant. This made him popular with SRs who welcomed the experience and responsibility, particularly as he was always willing to back up in case of difficulty.

The majority of his operating sessions were spent in the coffee room of the operating theatre, where he read and chatted amiably until the SR had completed the difficult procedures, after which he would depart for a local independent sector hospital where he had a thriving private practice.

Y took a ward round once a week, during which he would poke at an occasional abdomen and inspect stitches. This was his only appearance on the ward in the normal course of events, but he still took offence at being challenged (not unreasonably) to identify himself by a nurse who had been employed on the ward for some four months. The notes trolley did not accompany a Y ward round – a diagnosis list was all that he required – and the house officer had to be on guard that the round did not slip past without his or her knowledge. In general it took less than ten minutes to complete, after which Y would stop for a coffee with sister 'A' who was a personal friend. Junior medical staff were not welcome at this break.

The Senior Registrar at the time of my attachment to this unit was an ambitious, highly intelligent and, I felt, rather ruthless man, who had a wide social network of people upon whom he had operated. He was, on the other hand, a good surgeon who kept well up to date, and was involved in cancer research, about which he cared very much. His manner with patients was kind and considerate, and contrasted with his cool attitude to the rest of the staff.

The Registrar was pleasant, easygoing but relatively new to the rotation and consequently lacking in experience. This led to indecision and prevarication which at times left the house officers with a feeling of insecurity. As his appointment was as short-lived as that of the house officers, he did not feature largely in the culture of the organisation.

House officers. At any one time one of the HOs would be attached to the hospital orthopaedic unit, leaving two attached to the general surgical team. Because of tradition, this meant that the HOs worked a one-in-two rota (108 hours a week). The registrar and senior registrar also worked on a one-in-two basis but were only required to be present in the hospital on emergency take nights, or if called in for assistance by the house officers.

What are the motivations of doctors below the level of consultant? The description given by Handy of the self motivated individual in the large organisation does not apply to them since they have little in the way of power and their positions are far from secure, yet they do have the prospect of work, easily found, within their profession. Far the most likely explanation for their tolerance of their conditions is ambition: the prospect of a future position and of ultimately becoming consultants themselves provides motivation that outweighs the discomforts of the job at hand.

Latent organisational structure

I would like now to try to illustrate the manner in which, I perceive, things really worked on this unit. Although I did not analyse the reasons for it at the time, I was aware of the fact that the ward I knew was quite different from the one that I had expected. It was a far easier and more relaxed place in which to work than would be anticipated from the rigid and disciplined hierarchy outlined above. On reflection, I am aware that the positive feelings that I retain for the unit relate almost exclusively to my time on Ward 2, and that the culture of this ward had a noticeable spill over into the function of the rest of the unit. The situation as it really was can only be understood by introducing the leading nursing actors.

Nursing actors

Sister A (Ward 1) was in some respects an appropriate accompaniment to *X*'s view of how a ward should be run, as she was strict and disciplinarian with her staff, although less so with herself. The model of the ward as a bureaucratic pyramid fitted Ward 1 in fact as well as in theory. This disillusioned many of the nursing staff who came to work on the ward, and many left after only brief spells. As a consequence the ward was quite frequently short staffed, particularly with regard to state registered nurses (SRNs) capable of taking charge in *A*'s absence.

A's relations with the junior medical staff were thorny to say the least. Had she drawn the hierarchy in Diagram 2.3, I feel sure that HOs would have been placed below ward sisters with a heavy, controlling black line bearing down upon the box! Socially, *A* was close to the absentee consultant *Y*, and she was inclined to use his proxy 'opinions' to enhance her personal power. As these were never confirmed or reinforced by *Y* himself, such attempts at manipulation tended to be ignored.

Sister B (Ward 2) was probably the key player in this scenario. She was the sort of person who never really looked busy but had invariably finished all of the work. In contrast to *Sister A* who tended to alienate the staff she worked with, *Sister B* had managed to retain four or five first-class SRNs, any of whom had the ability to be a ward sister in her own right. This second line of 'lieutenants' meant that the running of the ward was fluent from one shift to the next.

On Ward 2 staff relations were excellent – probably the best of any ward I have ever worked on. Access to *Sister B* was open to any member of staff, whatever grade. Her office was used essentially as a common room, and the morning break was an established ritual of coffee and toast to which all members of staff were welcome. It may seem a little strange to attach significance to a coffee break, but this was the most visible sign of the way that Ward 2 functioned. It remains the only ward on which I have ever seen every member of staff, from the cleaner to the consultant, share their morning coffee as a matter of course. In the course of the day's routine, there was very little conflict, nor was there rigid adherence to tasks defined as being the responsibility of a specific person. As a result, when it came to preparing for X's ward rounds each afternoon, collection of results and X-rays was done by whoever was available at the time. This led to an atmosphere in which the ward round was largely an exercise in humouring X – if he went away thinking that his strict style of 'leadership' was producing good results, then everybody was happy.

Taking this into account I have massaged the original diagram of the ward hierarchy to produce the picture shown in Diagram 2.4. Ward 1 remains a rigid bureaucratic structure, but Ward 2 is an 'all channel' group which is now disproportionately large with respect to the rest of the unit. The HOs are now within this grouping to reflect our attachment to this sentient group, while the registrar hovers on the edge. In the diagram bold lines represent strong links and lighter lines weaker links of power and control. The senior registrar and consultants retain a semblance of the original medical hierarchy, but they are removed from the main body of the staff. The power of the Ward 1 bureaucracy is further diminished by its frequent reliance on Ward 2's reserve of expertise to bail it out of difficulty when short of staff.

I should emphasize that this represents the situation in routine circumstances. In emergencies it was notable that the pattern of behaviour which took over was far closer to the original design. This is consistent with the observation that in other organisations the authoritarian model is more effective at rapid responses. It was also interesting to see the behaviour of the medical staff at such times; X was reasonable and helpful, and would not lay blame for mistakes at the doors of his junior staff, Y would be available and cheerful even in the middle of the night, but the senior registrar would become surly and slightly vindictive – if a patient died he would occasionally apportion blame to his juniors.

Thus, the unit had a quite different *modus operandi* from that which appeared to be operational at a casual glance, but it was clear that this negotiated order had a second line of defence in the form of a more rigid hierarchy for dealing with crises.

Coda '. . . resource power has no potency.'

I spent four months attached to this unit with its peculiar blend of formal and open leadership, tolerating the sarcasm of Mr X, whom I had once considered a tyrant but had now found to be an anachronism, humoured by his staff. After two months, however, it was announced that the unit was to close on the very day that my colleagues and I moved on to our next

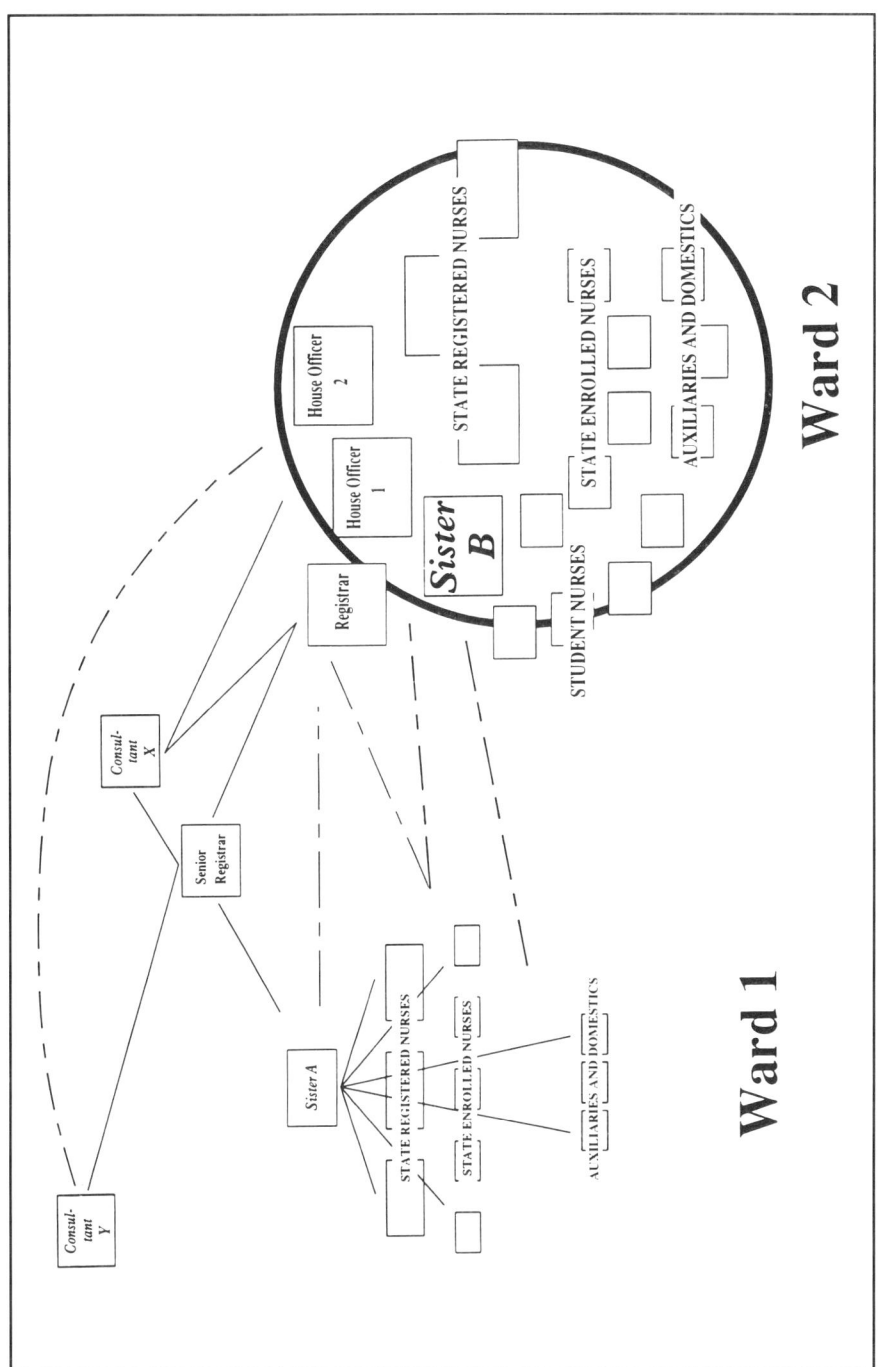

Diagram 2.4   The latent hierarchy

posts. The news seemed to irritate Y who took it as a personal insult, but for X it was devastating. He became visibly depressed and we were all touched by the pathos of a stubborn and difficult man brought low. I realized that I had become genuinely fond of him. There was no question that the unit had been substantially less busy than others in the same hospital; it was well known that the waiting time for a routine operation on Wards 1 and 2 was less than two weeks whereas other wards had lists of up to six months. X and Y, however had not sought to change the pattern of case distribution through the hospital, allowing the professorial unit to take the lion's share of the cases.

It can of course be argued in systems terms that the consultants had failed in a survival task – to maintain the supply of inputs – but in truth it illustrated the change being wrought in the NHS that continues in the current operative reforms. Both position and resource power are coming to have a stronger influence over once unassailable hospital consultants, and their colleagues (ie the professorial surgical unit in this case) may be more concerned with protecting their own interests.

The bureaucratic model that I envisaged initially was not only wrong internally, but was not the isolated and autonomous system that it seemed to be either. X's image of himself at the head of an independent clinical unit was wrong on both counts.

Case Study 2: The negotiated order in a gynaecological theatre

A Registrar

Editors' introduction
The context for this Case Study is a particularly interesting one in that the gynaecological theatre unit studied is in effect a 'staging post' for important operations to be carried out on patients. In such a unit, behavioural interactions between staff and patients are minimal compared to most other clinical units in a hospital. In these circumstances, the reward system or positive feedback on what is being achieved is predominantly inter-professional and not patient-to-professional. As the case study unfolds, the fact that the transitory nature of a patient's stay in the theatre unit for a technical procedure caused uncertainty about what constituted the primary goal of the unit, becomes apparent.

The study is set at a time when the strengthening of the general management function was being discussed but had not yet been implemented (Department of Health and Social Security, 1983). One of the recommendations of Griffiths was to appoint a general manager at unit (hospital) and other levels in the organisation in order to try to concentrate accountability for actions and efficiency in one person. A point for debate, with respect to this Case Study, is whether a reinforced general management function would have changed the dynamics of how this theatre unit functioned. This seems unlikely, given the nature of the decisions that had to be taken, often at short notice. As this Case Study shows, the resultant decisions were largely derived from a multitude of negotiations between different professionals using varied sources of power in order to get things done. The dominant coalition of professionals involved in the more important decisions also varied depending on the acuteness and nature of the problem. However, a core group of professionals tended to be members of the dominant coalition on most occasions, and this contributed to the stability of the functioning of the unit. The value of a respected enrolled nurse as a permanent member of staff in promoting stability should also be noted.

Organisational perspectives: while, in common with most of the Case Studies in this book, the writer draws on a combination of conceptual approaches to explore relationships in the gynaecological theatre, the most central part of the analysis relies on notions of different types of power (Introduction, p.23–4) and the ways in which they contribute to the emergence of a negotiated order (Introduction, p.29). These perspectives help to explain how the two separate hierarchies of doctors and nurses worked together in the theatre and provide an excellent example of how the formally less powerful members of an organisation can use their positions to exercise disproportionate influence on its functioning.

The Case Study

This Case Study describes the formal and informal organisation of an operating team in the gynaecological theatre of a large teaching hospital. Seen through the eyes of one of the members of the team, its main focus is on the role of bargaining between doctors and nurses in establishing viable and lasting working arrangements. The organisation is described as it was in the early 1980s and so there will be some differences from the present time in terms of formal National Health Service management structures.

The hospital was old and sprawled over a large site but the gynaecology unit, in which the theatre was located, was housed in a recently refurbished building. This was some distance from the maternity unit with which it had close links and where the medical staff spent much of their time. The senior medical and nursing staff had some input into the design and internal layout of the unit.

Management structure

The formal management structure is shown in a simplified form in Diagram 2.5. It can be seen that there was a well-defined management line down from regional management, through district and unit management, to the nursing officer tier. The nursing officers managed the sisters, who in turn managed the nursing staff. The place of the medical staff in this formal structure is not quite so clear. Some doctors were employed by the Regional Health Authority, but the vast majority, including the consultant staff were district employees. The ancillary staff were managed through the unit.

From Diagram 2.5 it would appear likely that the Nursing Officer (Gynaecology Unit) would have a key role in the organisation but this was not so. The organisation would have functioned quite adequately without her. The explanations for this are partly historical and partly personal. This individual had previously worked in the general medical unit of the hospital as a ward sister. She was one of a cohort of senior nurses who were encouraged to go into management with restructuring of nurse management following the Salmon Report in the early 1970s. Some very experienced, established senior nurses were channelled into management partly as career progression and partly because they would be able to command more appropriate financial rewards. Unfortunately, some of these nurses, of whom the Gynaecology Unit Nursing Officer was one, found a management post without direct responsibility for patient care less satisfying than ward management and discovered that they were not well-suited to management away from the front line. In the present instance this meant that the Nursing Officer was someone who, although she was in a position of authority, had no real power or influence.

The actors and the dominant coalition
The people in the organisation consisted of the medical staff, nursing and ancillary staff and patients. Both the medical staff and the nursing staff fitted the traditional hierarchical structures. These are shown in Diagram 2.6. It should be noted that the line of authority runs vertically through the individual hierarchies and that there is no formal management connection between. The link at that time was at district management level. Within the gynaecology unit, and especially during surgery, certain individuals perceived, wrongly, that they had authority over others in a different hierarchy.

The dominant coalition in the organisation consisted of the two nursing sisters and *Consultant A*. These were the people to whom one would look in times of crisis. Depending on the nature of the crisis *Consultant Anaesthetist C* might join the dominant coalition, as might another

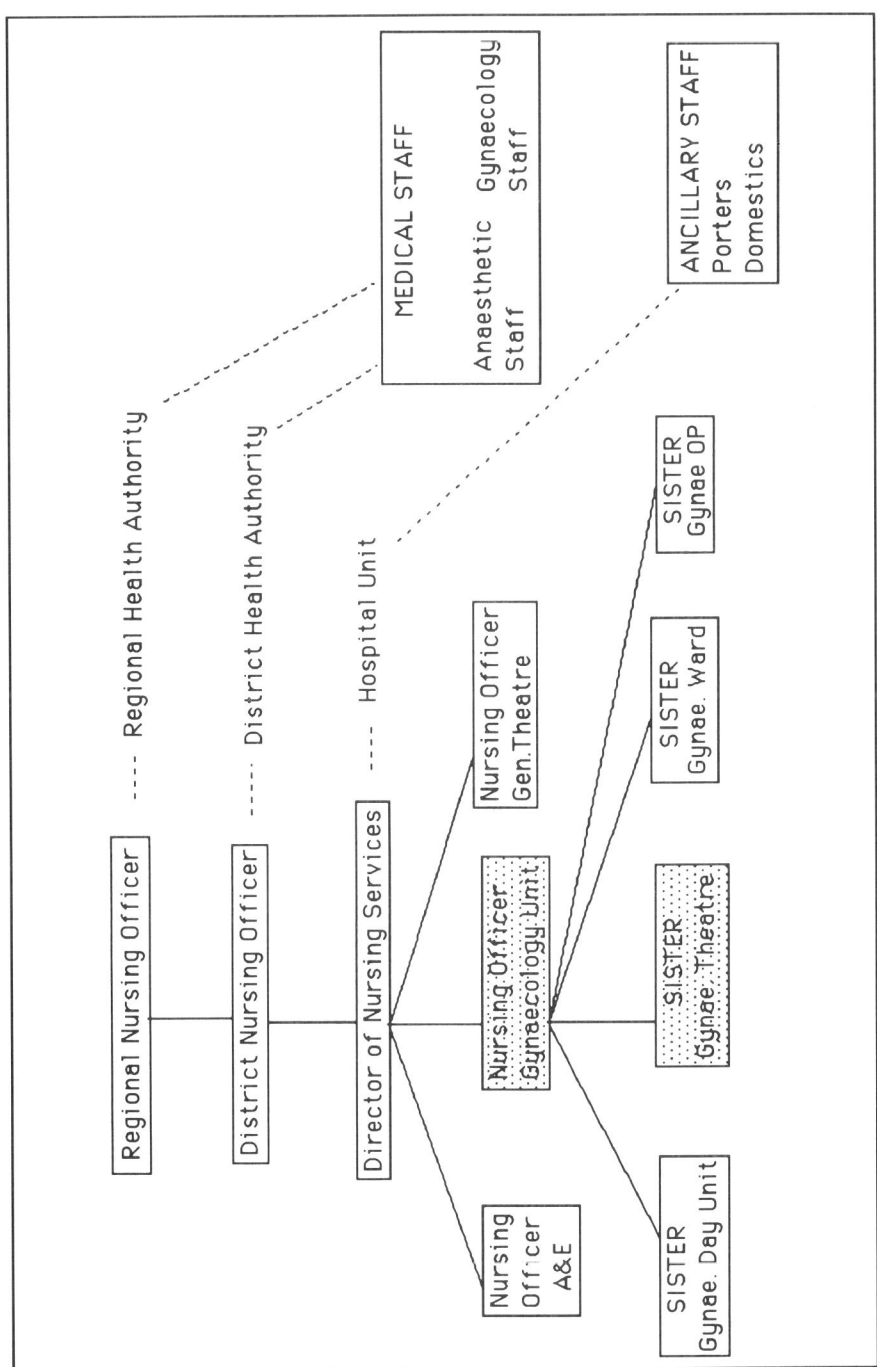

Diagram 2.5 The management structure of the gynaecological theatre

NURSING STAFF	MEDICAL STAFF	
	GYNAECOLOGY	ANAESTHETICS
Nursing Officer *(Gynae. Unit)* Sister X Sister Y Staff Nurses × 1–3 Student Nurses × 2–4 Enrolled Nurse ANCILLARY STAFF Orderly Cleaners Porters	Consultant A Consultant B Consultants ×3 Registrars × 4 Senior House Officers × 6 Pre-Registration House Officer Medical Students × 4	Consultant C Associate Specialists × 4

Diagram 2.6 Staff hierarchies in the gynaecological theatre

gynaecologist, *Consultant B*. These individuals tended to look to one another in different combinations depending on the task or problem involved.

The principal actors in the dominant coalition will be described in a little more detail.

Consultant A was consultant in administrative charge of the Obstetrics and Gynaecology Unit and he also held a university appointment. He was a very tall man and would physically dominate any group. Much of his professional life had been spent in a very senior position abroad. On his return to the United Kingdom, he firstly expected the rigid hierarchical medical structures which he remembered from his training days to have been preserved and, secondly, he brought back with him a rather 'colonial' attitude to his subordinates. He had an international reputation for his particular interest within gynaecology and was much in demand as a visiting lecturer and examiner. This, and his involvement with his Royal College meant that he was often abroad.

Consultant B was the second consultant gynaecologist. She deputised for *Consultant A* and was also respected for expertise and competence, but she did practise fairly traditional and possibly rather old-fashioned techniques which led to some friction with junior staff, particularly male Senior Registrars.

Sister X was the more senior of the two sisters. She was very experienced and was much respected by the medical and nursing staff alike. The nursing staff appreciated the way in which she protected their interests at times of possible conflict. However, she worked closely with *Consultant A* and the junior medical staff were aware that any misdemeanour on their part might be reported back to him. It was also apparent that while she would happily assist consultant staff in theatre, particularly *Consultant A*, she did tend to avoid assisting less experienced operators and would direct an inexperienced nurse to take this role. This was disappointing as the junior staff would have benefited from her expertise but it was not resented and she was well liked.

Sister Y was also popular. She had a big family and had trained as a mature entrant to nursing. Her promotion through the ranks had been encouraged and supported by *Consultant B*. Although *Sister X* and *Sister Y* were approximately the same age, *Sister Y* had been in the post for a relatively short time. Her experience outside nursing probably compensated for her relative lack of experience in it. She was excellent at her job and the best person to have around in an emergency.

Consultant Anaesthetist C was a female consultant who was greatly respected by all staff for her clinical competence and commonsense. Each day a different gynaecologist operated and each day had its own anaesthetist. *Consultant C* was consulted for advice on difficult cases by the other anaesthetists and gynaecologists on days other than her own. In addition junior staff would ask informally for advice on post-operative and other medical problems outwith theatre.

These principal actors had a stability and permanence within the organisation. The others, even although some were permanent staff, seemed much less important. The junior medical staff were on short-term appointments and the junior nursing staff moved on quickly, often for promotion. The enrolled nurse had been working there for many years. Student nurses and medical students spent only a month or two there at a time.

Obviously, from the individual patient's point of view she herself was one of the principal actors during her operation – perhaps even the 'star of the show' if her condition was particularly interesting or unusual or the operation technically difficult. However, from the organisation's point of view, each patient's appearance was very brief and, though a supply of patients was essential to ensure that the organisation could function, any group of women with the appropriate gynaecological problems would have done.

Tasks of the organisation

The primary task of the gynaecology theatre was to perform gynaecological surgery. This was what the organisation had to do in order to survive. There were two main mission tasks of the organisation: firstly, that of training nursing and medical staff, pre- and post-qualification, and secondly that of devising and refining new surgical techniques, which might be termed research and development. Ideally, improving the outcome for the patient should have been implicit within the definition of the primary task but it was more likely to have been an additional mission task.

The organisation as an open system

The organisation of the gynaecological theatre as an open system is illustrated in Diagram 2.7. Patients who required gynaecological surgery came from the community, either referred to outpatients by their general practitioners or presented as emergencies to the Accident and Emergency department, directly or as general practitioner referrals. They were admitted to one of the wards and transferred to theatre for surgery. A second input was medical and nursing students and junior doctors, the third input was instruments and procedures, and the skill of the operators can be seen as the fourth. The processes in the centre of the diagram in which inputs were transferred into output consisted mainly of surgical treatments. Training was also a fairly important part of the process and it is interesting to note that much of the input, namely junior doctors and student nurses undergoing training, accounted for a large proportion of the actors. The research and development function of the process was fairly small and ranged from a trial of a new type of surgical glove to an individual surgeon trying to perfect a particular technique.

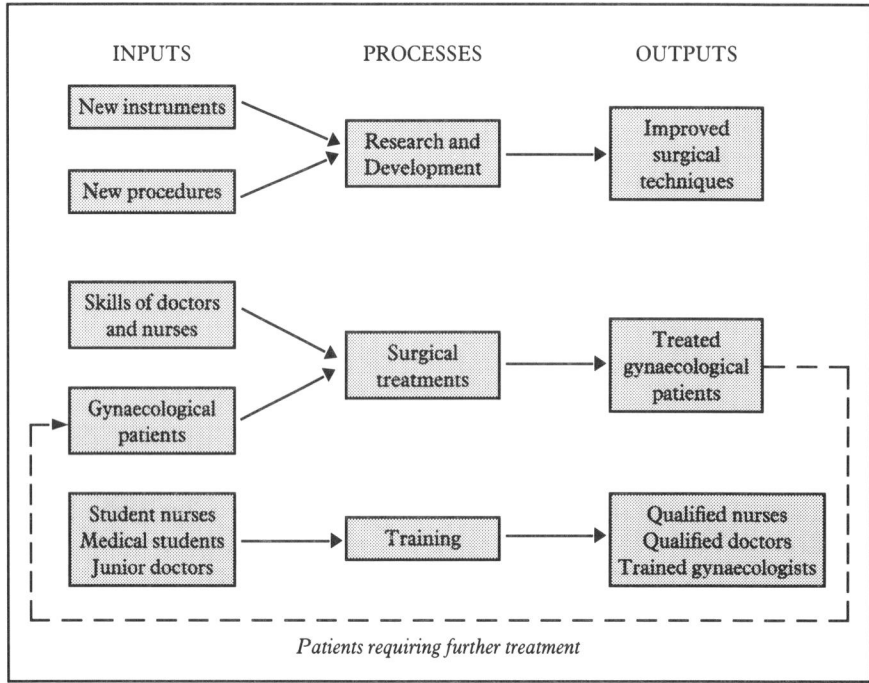

Diagram 2.7   The gynaecological theatre as an open system

The outputs were directly related to the inputs. The main output was certainly 'treated gynaecological patients'. It would be naive to say that this always meant 'cured' patients. Whilst some were fully cured as a result of the treatment, many were not. Some procedures were ameliorative rather than curative and others were investigative rather than therapeutic. Patients returned to the ward to recover and were then discharged to the community either to the care of their general practitioners or perhaps to return to the outpatient clinic, and possibly to re-enter the system! The training function was part of the production of qualified nurses and doctors, and of trained gynaecologists. Improved techniques and the use of better products may have resulted from the research and development function.

Power and authority in the gynaecological theatre

The medical and nursing staff made up two parallel hierarchical structures. *Consultant A* had authority over the medical staff. His power was of several sorts but the main one was position power. His role as consultant in administrative charge allowed him some resource power. He was the link between the gynaecological unit and the management groups in the hospital. Most would acknowledge his expert power. There was no doubt that he also had personal power based on his strong character and dominating presence. As a result of this combination of different kinds of power he was able to influence people and their behaviour well beyond the limits of his legitimate authority. For example, if there was a delay in a porter coming to theatre and a patient was awaiting transfer from the table to a trolley, he would instruct anyone who appeared to him to be available to lift the patient. No one refused but it was not part of anyone else's job to do heavy lifting like this.

Sister X had authority over the nursing staff. She had position power, expert power and personal power and used them all in different circumstances.

The levels at which the interactions between the two hierarchies and the negotiations took place is of interest. To help understand this the characteristics of some of the supporting actors need to be outlined. There were three other male, middle aged consultants and, as far as their role in the organisation was concerned, they were indistinguishable. The senior registrars who typically stayed for between twelve and eighteen months were usually male and invariably ambitious. The registrars and senior house officers were in the unit for between six months and one year. Some were training as specialists and others as general practitioners. Their experience formed a continuum and there was no such thing as a typical registrar or senior house officer. The house officer stayed only two months

– doing fairly menial routine tasks, regardless of his or her skill. Staff nurses were usually recently qualified and were gaining experience before moving on for promotion. The enrolled nurse was a stabilising influence. She was competent, happy with her job, and with its limits. She usually worked with the anaesthetist although she was an excellent scrub nurse. Student nurses came to this theatre near the end of their training. While some were interested in the work, others were not.

Motivation of the actors

The different groups certainly shared the same commitment to the primary task of providing good treatment but their motives and their dedication to the mission task varied. The senior nursing staff were involved in teaching and training the junior nurses, but they saw it as equally important to make certain that a list started and finished on time; this would ensure that everyone got off duty punctually (a goal which in the nurses' view might have been defined as a legitimate additional mission task of the organisation). They were aware that the managers would also be pleased as no overtime or entitlement to time off in lieu would be incurred. Some nursing staff did have loyalty to the organisation if, for example it had been their training school. The motives of the medical staff partly depended on the position of the doctor in the hierarchy. A consultant post in the NHS, which is a career grade, is usually a job for life and this may lead to loyalty and a commitment to the organisation. The consultants were committed to the primary and mission tasks and also to maintaining their positions of power. The junior medical staff, however, had different motives. They were working there to obtain training and qualification and the all important 'good reference'. Their loyalty to this particular organisation would not be great.

Negotiation and bargaining

As has been indicated, *Consultant A* had power far beyond that which derived from his position alone. He dominated the theatre even when he was not operating. All were aware of his likes and dislikes and if new medical staff did not quickly learn what they were, they were soon put in the picture by one of the sisters. His power over the other consultants was illustrated by his tendency to arrange to take one of his patients to theatre on someone else's list if he thought there was a space. If he wanted to operate at a particular time or on a particular day he would expect other consultants (but not *Consultant B*) to rearrange their lists to accommodate him. His dominant position defined the context for much of the other negotiation between the staff of the theatre behind the scenes.

Negotiation was most common between the registrars and the sisters. The sisters were in the stronger position. For example, daytime operating lists started at 9am and were due to finish by 5pm with a lunch break around 12.30. This theatre was also used for emergency cases and it remained open and staffed until 9pm, after which time cases had to be taken to the main theatre which was geographically separated from the unit. Such emergency cases were generally fairly straightforward and within the capabilities of the juniors. They were urgent cases in the sense that they had to be dealt with soon after admission rather than emergencies of a life and death kind. An example is the evacuation of the retained products of conception following an incomplete miscarriage. This operation should be carried out with some urgency in order to avoid the risk of further haemorrhage and to lessen the risk of infection. Gynaecological units with no dedicated emergency theatre adopt different approaches to this problem, but this unit had no defined policy and there was much bargaining and negotiating involved in fitting cases in. Registrars finishing off a consultant's list would take each other's emergency cases but certain anaesthetists did not like this. The registrars negotiated with nursing staff to be allowed to take patients to theatre in the early evening, at say 7pm, with promises of working quickly so that the nurses could clean theatre and get off duty on time. They would sometimes promise not to spend time teaching or supervising senior house officers in case this slowed things down. Inevitably it was easier to negotiate with some nurses than with others. Although the consultants were not involved in this negotiation, their names were often quoted. After 9pm cases had to be taken to the main theatre suite where delays caused by emergency cases from other specialties taking priority, unfamiliar equipment and staff and the distance from the maternity unit made the whole procedure rather inconvenient. Junior staff preferred not to operate there but consultants hated it. Perhaps they disliked having unfamiliar nursing staff who might not acknowledge their power. A registrar taking a slightly more complicated case to this theatre had to cope with the additional worry of having to ask a consultant to come in and help.

Formal rewards and sanctions within this organisation were limited, but unofficial ones were common and related to some of the negotiation and bargaining. Rewards were confined to praise and good reports given to staff, the reports being mainly for medical and nursing students. Good references were the formal rewards for junior doctors and praise from a senior colleague was an additional valued reward. Interestingly, patients rarely thanked theatre staff. They would thank their consultants and leave chocolates and flowers for the ward staff but the theatre staff were usually forgotten. Unofficial rewards were also important. An operating list which started on time and ran smoothly might result in such rewards being provided for the doctors and everyone else, by the nursing staff. Some lists were planned in such a way that a junior was expected to start with one or two minor cases before the consultant arrived half an hour later. If the list started late, the consultant would arrive ready to walk on in his leading role only to find the stage still occupied by the supporting cast. This made everyone cross, coffee breaks and even lunch might be delayed. If, however, things ran smoothly people felt good and the reward of toast would arrive with the coffee. Registrars who performed to the sisters' satisfaction might be rewarded with appropriately sized theatre wear and even personal footwear! For female staff in particular decent theatre wear is a worthwhile reward. As nurses started their period of duty before doctors, they had the first choice of the communal theatre wear. An unfortunate registrar, already feeling unsure of herself, was likely to find herself wearing a voluminous dress and shoes which pinched! Trivial rewards could assume some importance. *Consultant B* changed in the male changing room, whereas all the other female medical staff, including *Consultant C*, changed with the nurses. This 'privilege' may have been negotiated in the past.

The negotiated order varied in its stability. It was stable in that *Consultant A* headed the organisation. The remaining members of the dominant coalition followed and the other medical staff and nursing staff fitted together rather like jigsaw pieces below them. Although the pattern might have varied depending on the particular situation and on the individuals in post at the time, the negotiated order was sufficiently stable to allow continued survival of the organisation.

Conclusion

This organisation had no difficulty in achieving its primary task of a sufficient throughput of treated patients to justify its survival. The extent to which the mission tasks of training and research were achieved is, perhaps, less easy to assess given the open-ended nature of success in these areas. Nevertheless, cohorts of junior doctors were trained and research was carried out. The negotiated order which has been described in this case study was clearly a key factor in achieving working arrangements which satisfied important needs of all the main groups of actors in ways which were also consistent with the effective functioning of the gynaecological theatre. The formal NHS management structure and medical and nursing hierarchies in the theatre were common to almost all similar medical units at the time. This case study has demonstrated, however, that such structures are only part of the story and that to understand fully such organisations it is essential to look behind their outward face to the actual patterns of relationships which exist at any one time, and that such negotiated orders are likely in many ways to be unique to each different unit.

Case Study 3: Power and influence in a School Health Service Clinic

A Clinical Medical Officer

Editors' introduction

The setting for this Case Study is in neither a general practice nor a hospital firm but in the 'third arm' of the NHS, the community health services. In analysing the presence and nature of power and authority in this situation, it is important to be aware of the difficulties of career structure for doctors working in the community child health service. Although the 'well baby', developmental and immunisation clinics of this service (ie prevention and surveillance in young children) were brought under the umbrella of the NHS in 1974, there has subsequently been continuous discussion and debate about how best their functions should be organised. The Court Report published in 1976 recommended that all aspects of child health care, whether curative or preventive, should be dealt with wholly in general practice, perhaps by one of the partners in the practice who had undertaken some additional training in these aspects (Committee on Child Health Services, 1976). At the time, general practice as a whole did not subscribe to the view of the Report, but some GPs have always provided all forms of acute and preventive child health care and increasingly so in recent years.

There has been some concern, therefore, that community child health clinics provide duplicate care. As a consequence, the career structure and status for doctors working in community child health has been uncertain. This is exemplified in this Case Study by the transient or part-time nature of the involvement of the Clinical Medical Officers. There is therefore both a relative lack of authority and commitment, compared with that of hospital consultants or principals in general practice, which may explain in part the relinquishment of power to a junior member of the staff in the clinic described. As the study unfolds, however, other reasons for this will be become apparent.

Organisational perspectives: the main tools of analysis used in this case study are based on the concepts of action (Introduction, pages 28–9) and power (Introduction, pages 23–4). The author's use of the concepts of different kinds of power is particularly illuminating in illustrating the potential of what have been described as 'lower participants' in organisations (Mechanic, 1962) to achieve power far greater than their formal role in an organisation would warrant. In particular, this example supports Mechanic's hypotheses on the power lower participants can gain by making themselves irreplaceable, by occupying a central position in the structure, and by filling the vacuum created when higher ranking participants are unwilling to devote time to the proper discharge of their duties.

The Case Study

Legislation affecting the health of school children was introduced as far back as 1906, the basis for this legislation being the desire that ill health should not interfere with the learning process in schools. The emphasis was on prevention and the early detection of illness. Although the service was not included in the NHS at the time of its inception in 1948, remaining instead the responsibility of the Local Authority, the two services were amalgamated at the time of the 1974 reorganisation.

The school health service provides routine developmental assessments for all children up to the age of three and thereafter at 5, 10 and 15 years of age. The majority of these assessments are carried out by Clinical Medical Officers (CMOs) the 'school doctor', with the help of a school nurse (often referred to as Nitty Nora by children!). In addition to these assessments, CMOs also carry out immunisations and run baby clinics where parents can come and seek advice about their young children. A number of other health professionals are involved in the school health service, including health visitors, speech therapists, audiologists, physiotherapists, chiropodists and many others.

The Clinic

The particular child health clinic where I worked for two years was one of a number of similar clinics in the area, each one being situated within a community and serving the people and schools in that area. The clinic was housed in a two storey edifice built in the 1960s and was home to the Senior Clinical Medical Officer (SCMO), three CMOs, three health visitors, two school nurses, a physiotherapist, a speech therapist, an audiology technician, and four administrative staff.

Diagram 2.8 represents a simplified summary of staffing. Obviously there were Heads of all clinical specialties, the majority of whom worked at the largest clinic in the area (hereafter referred to as Central Clinic). The local clinic, where I worked, (hereafter known as Branch Clinic) was 15 miles away. There was a Senior Clinical Medical Officer (SCMO) at each local clinic who had overall authority over clinic staff. On the administrative side a Senior Administrative Assistant was responsible to the Head of Child Health at Central Clinic. Each local clinic had either an Higher

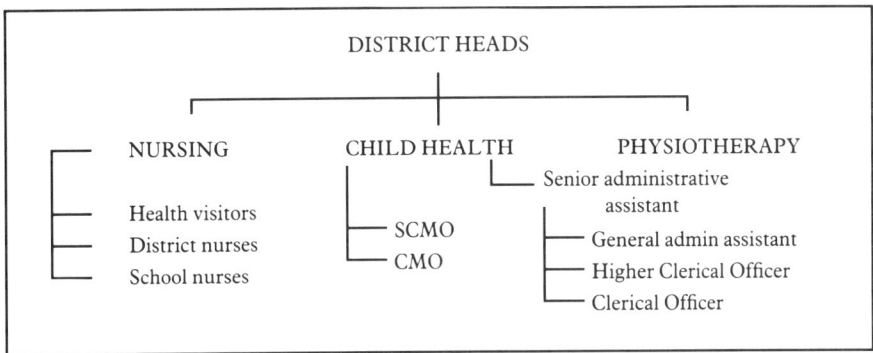

DISTRICT HEADS

NURSING   CHILD HEALTH   PHYSIOTHERAPY

Senior administrative assistant

Health visitors

District nurses   SCMO   General admin assistant

School nurses   CMO   Higher Clerical Officer

Clerical Officer

Diagram 2.8 The formal organisation of the School Health Clinic

Clerical Officer (HCO) or a General Administrative Assistant (GAA) heading the administrative section with Clerical Officers (COs) to help them.

Branch Clinic

Dr Thomas was the SCMO at Branch Clinic where I worked. She was a woman of 64 who had worked in the School Health Service all her life and remained fiercely dedicated to Branch Clinic and its clients. She had been widowed some years earlier and both her children lived in London, visiting only occasionally. Her job had thus become her life. Dr Thomas had been diagnosed as having cancer five years previously and despite operative intervention was becoming increasingly cachectic and unwell by the time I first started at Branch Clinic. Although all the clinic staff knew that Dr Thomas was suffering from a terminal illness, Dr Thomas herself was under the illusion that only her fellow SCMOs and the HCO at the clinic knew of her condition. Whenever Dr Thomas needed to take time off for medical check-ups she always told the CMOs that she was seeing the dentist! However the HCO could always be relied upon to broadcast the true story to all and sundry.

The other main body of staff at Branch Clinic were the administrative staff. They dealt with all the clerical work, made appointments for clients, supervised the domestic staff and generally organised the day-to-day running of the clinic. They were headed by the formidable Mrs Mac (thus known on account of her Scottish ancestry) who was an HCO. Beneath her were three COs, all of whom were teenage girls. Mrs Mac would switch from extolling their virtues to deriding them depending on her mood! It was Mrs Mac who was at the centre of the problems at Branch Clinic. She was a domineering woman in her 60's (nobody knew exactly what age!) who had been at Branch Clinic since it had been built and was known by us as the Führer. Although the dominant coalition at the clinic had been

Dr Thomas supported by Mrs Mac, at some point the situation had reversed itself and by the time I came to work at the clinic it was Mrs Mac who was effectively in charge despite Dr Thomas's formal authority. It was only on the rare occasions when Mrs Mac was away that Dr Thomas regained her rightful position. I was told by other staff at the clinic that prior to her illness Dr Thomas had always been firmly in the driving seat. However, around the time of her first operation Dr Thomas and Mrs Mac, who had always been very friendly towards one another, had had a major disagreement. Thus the true management structure at Branch Clinic was that shown in Diagram 2.9.

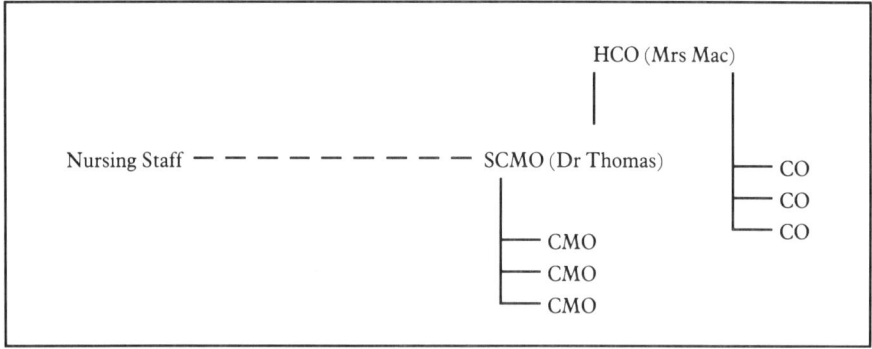

Diagram 2.9   The latent management structure at branch clinic

Mrs Mac and 'her girls' occupied a large office at the front of the clinic, one wall of which was glass and acted as the reception window for clients, whilst also affording Mrs Mac a bird's eye view of all the comings and goings of various staff. The 'girls' were expected to attend to any queries at the window regardless of what they were doing since Mrs Mac remained firmly in her chair in all but exceptional circumstances. The 'girls' worked at three separate desks arranged in front of Mrs Mac and no social talking was allowed except at coffee time, when one of the girls was despatched to make coffee for the merry band! During coffee breaks Mrs Mac generally became very friendly towards 'her girls' and would regale them with her opinions of the medical staff (not usually complimentary) whilst extolling the virtues of the doctor who was her current favourite.

Both Mrs Mac and Dr Thomas shared several things in common: neither of them trained their staff comprehensively, which led to problems if either of them was away. In the case of Dr Thomas, she dealt with all the special schools (ie those catering for children with special needs) herself and delegated all the routine school work. With her declining health, she was increasingly off work and the CMOs who had little experience of assessing children with special needs had to take over her clinics in the special schools, most of which we had never visited. In the case of Mrs Mac, she was involved in an accident soon after I joined in which she sustained injuries which kept her off work for around ten weeks. During that time all 'special referrals' (ie referrals to certain hospital specialists) were stockpiled since this was one of Mrs Mac's special tasks which none of the COs knew how to process. Both women, too, had adopted their desks as their own personal property. No-one ever occupied Mrs Mac's desk, even during her long sick leave, despite its position at the front of the office which was ideal for dealing with clients at the reception window. Similarly, her typewriter, which was superior to any of the others in the office, remained under its dust cover. Mrs Mac's desk was always locked in her absence and she held the only known key – the contents of her desk drawers were always much speculated upon by the junior doctors! Dr Thomas occupied the only purpose built medical room in the clinic in which there was an examination couch and various pieces of routine medical equipment. Although all the doctors were allowed to use this room for clinics, we could only do so when Dr Thomas was working away from the clinic. Even when she was only writing letters in her room the other doctors would have to use an alternative room in which to see their patients, even though many of these rooms were far from satisfactory for carrying out examinations.

The main problems at the clinic were due to Mrs Mac's constant sniping at certain doctors or nurses or at any staff for that matter – no-one was immune! This caused a lot of tension and unhappiness amongst staff. Mrs Mac liked to feel she was boss and was never happier than when sitting at her desk directing operations and watching everyone running around like headless chickens! She had a very dominant personality and was not averse to telling minor untruths. When giving instructions to doctors, she often implied that she was passing on information from Dr Thomas, when in fact Dr Thomas had no knowledge of the situation. For instance, if a referral to a consultant wasn't completed in the manner she favoured, Mrs Mac would often preface her remarks with a phrase such as 'Dr Thomas doesn't like things done like that ...'.

The bases of the power of the Higher Clerical Officer (HCO)

Thus the position at Branch Clinic was one where Mrs Mac was making most of the decisions concerning the running and service provision of the clinic. This was undoubtedly due in the main to Dr Thomas's declining health. Mrs Mac was known for her stubborness and would rarely back down without a full scale battle of words many of which were very unpleasant. Dr Thomas would often retreat in the face of such an argument, finding it easier to go along with Mrs Mac than oppose her.

Homans (1951) has said that all arguments involve an exchange of something for something in return and Dr Thomas was prepared to forego her position as leader of the dominant coalition for a 'quiet life'. Dr Thomas also aided and abetted Mrs Mac in many ways; for instance, she would not approve doctors' holiday leave until Mrs Mac had confirmed the arrangements were convenient, even though Mrs Mac had no real authority to veto doctors' holidays. Of course, Mrs Mac was in her element and always made a great show of checking through the clinic diaries before confirming that it was acceptable to take holidays.

There are a variety of categorisations of power and Mrs Mac possessed several possible sources which gave her the ability to influence others. Her mainstay was probably *coercive power*. Although she was only a small woman, she was a bully and her stinging personal attacks had left several members of staff in tears and created a tense atmosphere for weeks afterwards. Mrs Mac played a major role in the recruitment of clerical staff and it was noticeable that successive COs were all very similar – they tended to be teenage girls who were generally very quiet. This was in marked contrast to neighbouring clinics where COs were in the 25–35 year age bracket and much more outgoing. It seemed that Mrs Mac tended to favour young, naive girls whom she could easily dominate and could be relied on to support her views, often resulting in their uncharacteristic unhelpfulness towards disfavoured members of staff.

In addition to her coercive power, Mrs Mac had an element of *resource power*, since the greater her dislike for a particular member of staff, the more friendly she was with other members of staff. She would reward compliant medical staff by making them coffee half-way through clinic and generally treating them with the utmost of respect. However, as is often the case, resource power is not particularly popular, since no-one likes to acknowledge that they can be bought; when one of us was treated to coffee it was generally regarded with rueful embarrassment.

Mrs Mac had very little position or legitimate power though she did have a degree of expert power, albeit much less than Dr Thomas's. None of the clerical staff were cognisant with all the facets of her job, which made her indispensable in some respects. Certainly during Mrs Mac's sick leave things became chaotic, since much work had to be put on one side for her to do, and none of the girls was capable of deputising effectively for her. Mrs Mac certainly lacked personal power but had a degree of negative power since most incoming mail and messages came through her and she was often known to delay important messages when the mood took her. Negative power tends not to operate all the time and is manifest mainly in times of stress or frustration – Mrs Mac tended only to delay the messages of currently disfavoured staff.

Mrs Mac's various power bases allowed her to influence the staff of Branch Clinic. The crudest of her methods was coercion – manifest in the threat of a public argument. Since Mrs Mac had no real position power she had little recourse to rules and procedures. She used exchange methods to reward compliant behaviour. However it takes two to tango and, as the recipients of Mrs Mac's influence, we could have rejected or ignored it and battled with her. Mrs Mac was fortunate in that the staff at the clinic were generally compliant and disliked conflict. None of the CMOs worked full time – two of the CMOs also worked part time in general practice and were in fact awaiting full time GP posts, and I had a year's contract in order to gain experience in the community before beginning training in Public Health Medicine. In addition, Dr Thomas with her declining health greatly disliked conflict and was rarely supportive of medical staff when conflict did occur.

It has been shown how the power gained by Mrs Mac and the way she chose to use it adversely affected the operation of the clinic in a number of ways. In particular, it left specialist referrals unallocated when she was away, led to the recruitment of inexperienced and timid clerical officers and maintained the marginal status of the CMOs in the professional management of the clinic, so minimising any chance that they would act to tackle the problems arising from the increasing illness of the SCMO.

Fortunately, however, although there was often a degree of tension between Mrs Mac and the clinic doctors, this did not often affect the quality of service each doctor gave to her clients. In fact Mrs Mac regarded clients as a bit of a nuisance in that they interfered with the smooth running of the clinic. It was thus lucky that, apart from her responsibility for specialist referrals, she had very little to do with them, delegating that side of the job to her junior staff. Although the nature of the relationship between Mrs Mac and Dr Thomas was well known to others in the School Health Service, including the district Head of Administration at Central Clinic, no action was ever taken to resolve the situation. This was partly because both Mrs Mac and Dr Thomas were in their sixties and therefore would soon be retiring. Further, the consequences of Mrs Mac's ascendancy were not fully understood outside the clinic; both women were regarded as being good at their jobs and Branch Clinic was perceived as being run very efficiently.

Three months after I finished the job and shortly after her retirement, Dr Thomas died of cancer. Six months later, having told no one, Mrs Mac suddenly announced that she would be retiring at the end of the week and requested no leaving celebrations. She has never visited the clinic since.

Conflict

Introduction

Conflict is sometimes argued to be a natural and even essential part of organisational evolution and adaptation (see, for example, Peters, 1987). The first two studies in this section (Case Studies 4 and 5), however, deal with conflicts which have more to do with the failure of management to balance the demands of the different goals of treatment and training (and in one case, research) in the organisations concerned than with development. The third study (Case Study 6), in contrast, explores conflict in the context of a leadership struggle between two consultants and illustrates the unplanned character of the changes which were involved.

Case Study 4: Conflict in a Medical Firm

A House Officer

Editors' introduction
This Case Study graphically illustrates the dilemmas facing the newly qualified doctor on appointment to a pre-registration post in a hospital firm. In the early years of a doctor's career, appointments are short term in nature. The potential benefit for doctors is that they have the opportunity of gathering skills under supervision in a variety of clinical fields in the early phase of their careers. However, the tension and uncertainty that these short-term contracts create for the holders, with respect to perceived future employment, becomes readily apparent. The behaviour that this creates should not go unnoticed in a society in which there is a general movement, encouraged in the public sector by government, towards temporary or short-term employment contracts at all stages of careers.

Such newly qualified doctors feel an ambiguity in their role. They have responsible technical procedures to carry out for their patients at the same time as having to establish rapport with them. In the particular situation described, although feeling this responsibility, the young doctors were allowed little discretion in decisions about individual patients. Moreover, the juniors were involved in day-to-day administration of activities on the ward but appeared to have neither opportunities nor a forum for changing the situation for the better. It should also be noted that this Case-Study represents an example of a specialist firm within an institution (a teaching hospital) with multiple goals, two of which, treatment and care on the one hand and research on the other, create tensions for the young doctors involved.

In addition to the authority attributed to the consultants by the junior doctors concerned, they were also perceived as wielding power through the junior doctors' need to receive a reference at the end of the short-term appointment. Control was also exerted by the consultants through the use of intemperate language when problems occurred. Particularly interesting is the use of negative power by the house officers (HOs) as their response to the highly varied nature of the demands placed upon them within the different subsystems of this clinical firm. As a result, conflict was bound to occur. Points to note about the partial resolution described are: firstly, the gross nature of the signs of distress in the participants before the most sensitive of the higher ranking juniors stepped in with some simple remedies; secondly, in an age of general management, the dilemma and any measures taken to resolve it were considered to be solely within the clinical ambit; and thirdly, when the next new group of HOs started their six month posts in the firm, the more permanent members appeared not to have learned from the previous experience. A point to which we return in the 'Conclusion' is whether the disharmony of the kind found in this clinical firm could have been prevented by prior management training and, if so, at what stage or stages of a medical student's or doctor's career such training should have been introduced.

Organisational perspectives: the writer has drawn on several themes in organisational theory to construct this analysis and the Case Study illustrates clearly the value of an eclectic approach of this kind. The central problem confronting the organisation of pursuing simultaneously a number of different goals is brought out clearly by the use of a systems approach (Introduction, pages 25–6). This leads the writer to an analysis of the different subsystems related to these goals and to an examination of their incompatible elements. The use of an action perspective (Introduction, page 28–9) helps to explain the initial failure of the firm to grapple with the crisis emerging from the situation, while an understanding of human relations methods in management (Introduction, pages 26–8) helps to explain how the intervention of the registrar led to a temporary solution.

The Case Study

Every six months each medical firm in Britain is joined by the new 'house'. The 'house' comprises various numbers of junior and senior house officers. For the junior house officers (HOs), successful completion of the six month appointment is necessary for them to be fully registered as medical practitioners. Senior house officers (SHOs), already registered, move from firm to firm gaining specialised experience to help them to climb the long career ladder towards becoming clinical consultants. This study draws on some of the various contributions to organisation theory in order to describe some of the changes observed whilst working as a newly qualified medical house officer and part of the new 'house' within a specialist medical firm.

The structure and functions of the firm are first described using some of the principles which underly the systems theory of organisations. This is followed by a description of the conflict which arose within the firm following the change of 'house'. Because of the limitations of systems theory, some of the writings on action theory and neohuman relations have also been drawn upon in order to explain adequately the sources of conflict in the organisation. The study concludes by outlining how the difficulties within the organisation were resolved and, by using contingency theory, attempts to predict how future changes of 'house' may affect the organisation.

The organisation

The medical firm was based in a modern, busy, teaching hospital. As such, its main function (indeed, its primary survival goal) was to take ill patients and transform them to either cured patients, or patients whose symptoms had been relieved in some way. This action of transforming the patients involved a number of processes which are illustrated in Diagram 2.10. The unit was also a regional centre for the specialised management of patients with respiratory diseases and to function as this, it also had to provide a number of subsystems peculiar to that firm. These systems are shown in Diagram 2.11. These subsystems had to function adequately to ensure that the unit could move towards fulfilling its mission task, that is to have an international reputation as a centre of excellence for the management of patients with respiratory disease. The medical literature was full of research produced by the unit as a testament to their achievement of this mission goal.

Both the primary or survival goal (the correct treatment and care of patients) and secondary or mission goal (maintaining status as a centre of excellence) were met so successfully that there was a constant flow of referrals for treatment which provided a rich source of subjects to enter the other subsystems. The involvement of the other subsystems made the task of transforming the patients far more complex than in other units which do not have these subsystems.

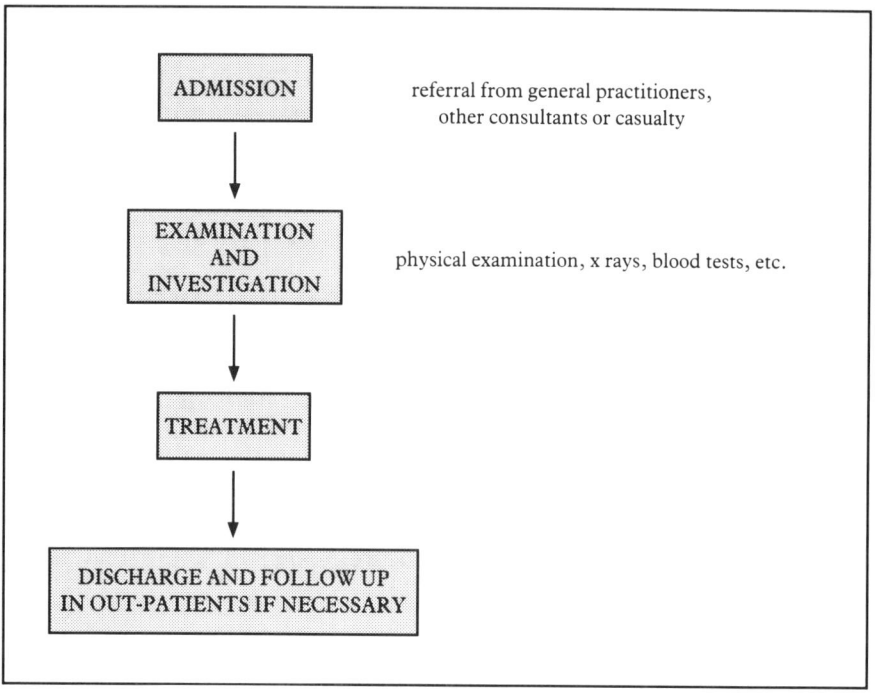

Diagram 2.10 Work flow in the medical firm

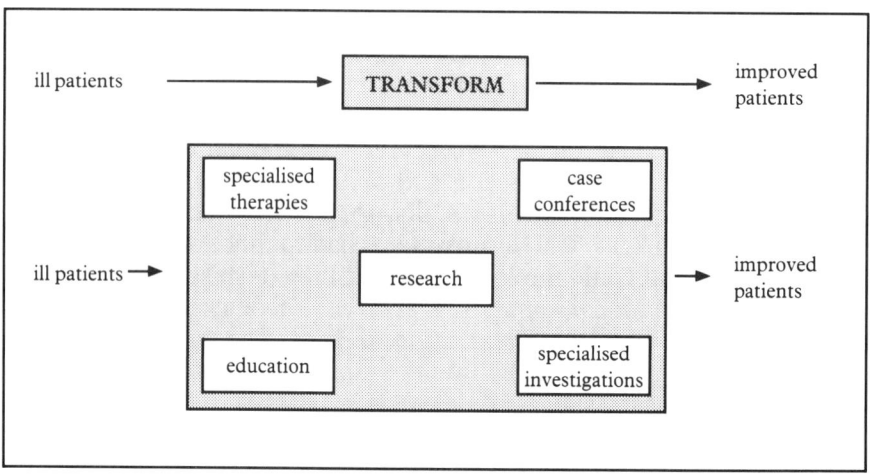

Diagram 2.11 Subsystems in the medical firm

The established structure

There were twelve doctors in the firm which had a clear hierarchical structure similar to many medical firms. This structure is summarised in Diagram 2.12.

There were four clearly defined and separate groups: the consultants; the senior registrar and the registrar; the research registrars; the house officers (SHOs and HOs). The consultants were the only permanent members of the team, each with differing involvement in the system and subsystems. *AB* acted as the leader of the firm, negotiating monies and promoting its reputation. *CD* had less involvement in the subsystem, whereas *EF*'s priority was research. Their role was to ensure attainment of the mission task.

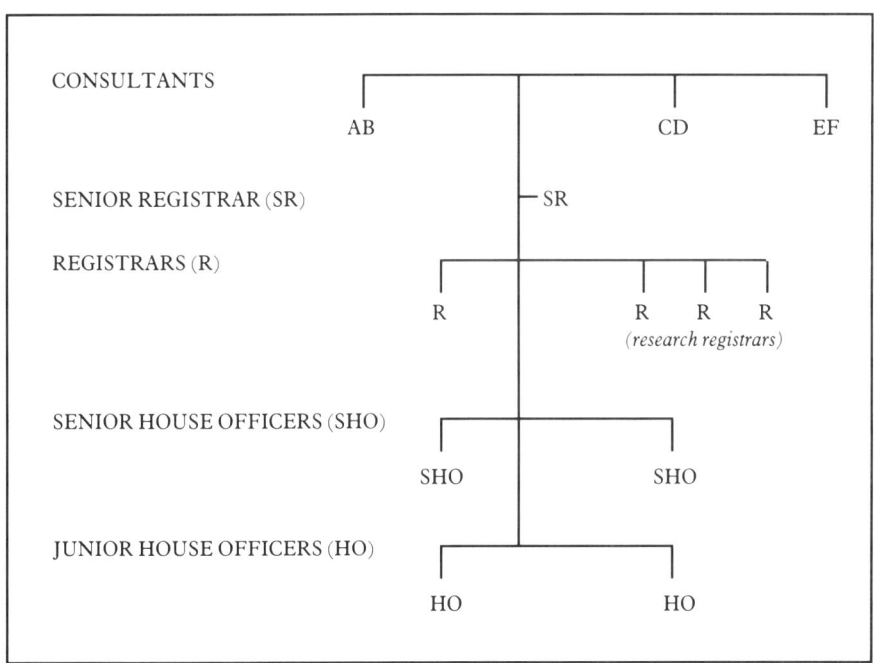

Diagram 2.12   The medical hierarchy

The senior registrar had a two year job contract with the unit and had been with the firm one year when the new 'house' arrived. The registrar joined the firm at the same time as the 'house' but was due to stay for one year in contrast to the SHOs and HOs whose contracts were for six months only. All of these were involved in all the systems but their main role was to manage the organisation such that the primary survival goal would not be jeopardised. The research registrars were only involved in the research subsystem and did not contribute to the core task in any way.

Every member of the 'house' (two HOs and two SHOs) was new to the firm. Also, we were all new to our positions. The SHOs had only just finished their pre-registration house year, and myself and the other house officer had only just qualified as doctors. As part of the 'house' we were responsible for the core task of the firm; admitting patients, organising and undertaking the appropriate investigations and then, following diagnosis, organising and administering treatment. We would then liaise with the nursing staff to organise the patients' discharge home and arrange their follow-up if necessary. Because of the complex nature of transforming these patients, the emphasis was on smooth and efficient organisation.

Authority and role discretion within the unit

As house officers, we were required to employ a degree of discretion in our diagnosis and treatment because we dealt with so many patients whose health status and health care needs varied from day to day. However, because we were inexperienced, this had potentially grave implications which could have jeopardised the survival goal of the unit and as a result, the consultants ensured that we were closely supervised. The SHOs, the registrar and the senior registrar were all responsible for our actions. In order to restrict our level of discretion there were a number of clinical protocols in place which we had to follow (such protocols are not common to all medical firms but involve fixed definitive rules concerning the investigation of patients). Any strategic decisions regarding individual patients were only made by the consultants. This, in addition to the protocols, ensured the dominance of what Rensis Likert has called a System One or exploitive authoritative approach to management, with centralised control (Likert, 1967).

The consultants asserted their power within the firm by using verbal threats; shouting and publically humiliating each member of the house. All three consultants were perceived as extremely impatient and bad tempered and if there were any problems, regardless of their magnitude, at least one would vent his anger by erupting with a torrent of verbal abuse, swearing at whoever appeared to be responsible. Needless to say, as inexperienced doctors working within such a busy and complex firm, the house officers found it especially difficult to maintain smooth organisation and we were subjected to these outbursts almost daily. Our future was wholly dependent on these consultants who would give approval for registration with the General Medical Council and whose references would secure us our future jobs. The consultants held this resource power and we lived in constant fear of being deprived of our admission ticket to a continuing medical career. The consultants were aware of this and regularly used it as a weapon with which to threaten us.

Conflict

As HOs, we found ourselves under constant pressure from the start of the job. There were a number of stresses peculiar to us as newly qualified doctors. We were undergoing a rapid process of socialisation into the medical profession and the role of a doctor rather than that of a medical student, but the responsibility, workload and long hours were difficult to come to terms with. Our personal primary survival task was to complete the six month appointment in a manner satisfactory to the consultants so that we would be approved for full registration. However, we shared the same mission task, namely to secure glowing references from the consultants which would guarantee our future success. Consequently, the consultants' power was unquestioned but in comparison, that of the SHOs, the registrars and the senior registrar was insignificant.

This led to a number of problems when dealing with the SHOs, in particular. Part of the problem was that the members of the 'house' had different expectations of the role of the SHO which had never been clearly defined. The SHOs saw themselves in a supervisory capacity in relation to us, and had legitimate power for this role. However, they found it difficult to assert their authority because we only paid heed to that of the consultants. It has been suggested that there are five major kinds of power in organisations: coercive, resource, position, expert and personal.

Given their lack of authority and the negligible power vested in their position, the SHOs had a number of alternative sources of power available to them which could have been useful in dealing with us. Their most valuable resource was their previous experience of coping with uncertainty and also as a potentially greater source of expert knowledge than the house officers. However, as time wore on their 'expert knowledge' did not materialise, nor did they appear to have an ability to cope with uncertainty; as a result we looked to the registrar and the senior registrar for these resources. The potential for the SHOs to use personal charismatic power was very limited as both the nurses and the medical staff felt them to be disagreeable individuals, lacking social skills. Because they did not have any of the resources we expected from them we felt that the SHOs would be more valuable if they were to share some of our heavy workload. The SHOs did not consider that such menial work was within their remit and continued to try, unsuccessfully, to assert their authority. They did this by trying to prove their expert knowledge by asking us to undertake additional esoteric tests on the patients. These apparently unnecessary tasks were seen to have no other purpose but to add further to our already excessive workload. In order to avoid this extra work, we started to marginalise the SHOs. We avoided discussing our patients with them, and if we needed help for the purposes of guiding patient care, we turned directly to the registrar or the senior registrar.

As time went on this conflict began to manifest itself within the completion of the core task. On ward rounds the consultants were disturbed to discover that the SHOs knew very little about their patients and the registrar was irritated at having to deal with problems which should have been adequately dealt with by them. Consequently, both these groups vented their irritation on these apparently incompetent SHOs. Unfortunately, we were often included as targets in the firing line. The result was poor communication and worsening morale. One of the junior doctors leaving the ward round in tears became a regular feature of the working day. This was disturbing to the whole unit.

Another source of conflict within the firm arose from the research subsystem. The work which it entailed for us led to considerable personal tensions; we were responsible for gaining patients' consent for research treatment trials and for giving the test treatments. The nature of randomised controlled trials necessarily means that a new treatment is being compared with a conventional treatment to investigate in a scientific manner which is the superior. That is to say, trials are carried out in circumstances of genuine uncertainty about the best treatment. Nevertheless, some new treatments at times involved discomfort for the patient and this led to feelings of role incompatibility between the doctor as carer, and the doctor as researcher which contributed further to the poor morale in the unit.

The nurses often shared our concerns and as a result of our common feelings we formed a sentient group with them. All trials have exclusion criteria which define circumstances in which patients should not be asked to take part in them and our approach was to err continually on the side of exclusion. We would collude to arrange for the terminally ill patients who were due for more research-orientated treatment to be discharged before the next ward round when their treatment plan would be determined. In the process of fulfilling the research trial protocol, we would ensure that patients and relatives were fully aware of the trial conditions, and we were careful not to convey any enthusiasm for the trial prior to seeking consent for inclusion. Resistance to inclusion in a trial by patient or relative was accepted without question as a reason for exclusion without further attempt at persuasion. Indeed, a hint of resistance by patient or relative was sometimes positively encouraged by the HOs.

The research limb of the organisation also contributed significantly to our already excessive workload; we were forced to undertake additional blood tests and investigations. We felt that the routine care of patients was most important and that research should have a lower priority. Hence many of these tests, which did not prejudice the assessment or direct care of the patient, were conveniently 'forgotten'. This worked for a while but the research registrars would constantly badger us for the tests so that it could only be a holding measure. These activities put the research subsystem into disarray. Recruitment to trials was low and research programmes were not being completed. The consultants were angry and irritable at seeing their mission task threatened. Needless to say, they vented their anger on us but we felt our actions were justifiable and did not change them. We became more depressed; it seemed we could do nothing right and I abandoned my personal mission task (achieving a high quality reference) and concentrated on surviving (simply to obtain the consultant's signature to enable full registration as a doctor to take place). Job satisfaction was minimal; we were surrounded by the apparent suffering of fellow staff who were subject to intense emotional demands to which we seemed to be contributing. There was a dreadful sense of futility pervading the lower ranks of the firm.

Unfortunately we were faced with another source of conflict; we were forced to prioritise our excessive workload. We seemed to be suffering from role overload, finding it difficult to be doctor, administrator and student. It was impossible to fulfil all roles to any level of excellence and as a result we gave the administrative tasks a low priority since they appeared to be less important than the others. A consequence of this was that patients' casenotes were poorly maintained; patients were often discharged without an immediate letter for their family doctor and many did not get the necessary arrangements for follow-up. These actions had more serious implications for the unit than many of the others; general practitioners complained to the consultants and often their queries could not be answered because of the inadequate casenotes. The out-patient clinics were in disarray and the quality of service provided by the medical unit appeared to be deteriorating.

The system was malfunctioning, and not only was the unit's mission task failing, but its survival goal was under attack. Relationships within the firm were appalling; the consultants were permanently irritable and angry and the rest of us were depressed and disillusioned. Everyone seemed to be venting their anger on the HOs and our inadequacies. We were becoming increasingly worried that we would not even achieve our minimal aim of getting positive references from the consultants; we thought we were doing everything we could (if not more) and still no one was satisfied. In retrospect it is clear that our perceptions of our role were different to those of our superiors. We were trying to be doctors, they wanted efficient ward clerks and pairs of hands to support the research function. Medical school had taught us that being a doctor was about treating patients; the organisational and research elements of being a doctor were new to us and as our contact with patients was limited to their in-patient care, we were under the impression that follow-up was 'someone else's job'. No one within the firm had explained to us the relevance of the research, communication or administration for the viability of the organisation, or more importantly for the continuing care of patients; they just shouted at us when things went wrong.

Resolution and negotiated order

It was the registrar who attempted to resolve some of the conflict. She was the more sensitive of the junior doctors above the HOs in the hierarchy and, in part, was responding to the continuing bouts of emotional display at the end of ward rounds. There was also pressure from the consultants to rectify the situation and this registrar was charged with the responsibility for general administration of clinical matters in the firm. She diagnosed poor communication as both a cause and a symptom of the situation and commenced treatment by encouraging us to communicate more actively with the SHOs. The other HO and myself had been sharing our work informally, and the SHOs had no formal system for sharing their responsibilities or our supervision. The registrar organised us to work in pairs, one SHO and HO to be jointly responsible for the male patients and the remaining HO and SHO to be jointly reponsible for the female patients. She made it clear to us that the HOs were to be directly responsible to their relevant SHO, who in turn was expected to help with the HO's workload.

As a result we started to have new working relationships. We traded our information and communication with the SHOs for help with our work. The SHOs no longer had to struggle to assert their authority and they appeared to become more aware of our needs through the increased interaction and sharing of problems and tensions. On busy days they would bring us biscuits or sweets to cheer us up. Although these were initially used as bribes, we all eventually became good friends. The registrar continued her interventions by offering a form of after care; whereas previously she had apparently worked in isolation, now she took on a new role as the juniors' team leader. She would round us all up for lunch and if we were too busy to leave the ward she would fetch us sandwiches and legitimise a work break for sustenance. We got to know her well as she would call in at the ward in the morning, and in the afternoon to see how things were going. As a result she got to know us all on a personal level and would listen to the reasons for our misgivings, worries and disillusionment. She gained our trust and gave us some feedback about our performance and why some aspects of it were unsatisfactory. We learned about the whole organisation and that treating the patients was just a small part of this great system.

Maslow's hierarchy of needs (Maslow, 1954) outlines the fact that the needs of an individual for survival must be satisfied before any self-actualisation can occur. Certainly in this unit, once someone had paid some attention to our needs for food, rest, friendship, and esteem, we started to get more out of our job. Ward rounds which had previously ended in tears, soon began to end in laughter and the consultants' intolerance became a predictable fact of life which was unlikely to threaten our survival goal. Our newly formed teams provided for far better patient care, and also released time so that we could allocate more time for administrative tasks. The unit's personnel were able to resume providing a high quality service approaching its mission task. Looking back, the issue of incompatibility with the research was not resolved in any explicit way but the problem did seem to dissipate. As we showed more awareness of the functions of the organisation and the wider role of the doctor, we became increasingly socialised into the culture of the unit and more accepting of the research subsystem. The feelings of role incompatibility therefore lessened. We continued to collude with the nurses in arranging for the terminal patients to go home before becoming involved in research treatments, but we were more ready to seek consent from other patients.

At the end of our six month appointment, the whole firm agreed that this had been an excellent 'house' and we all received good references. In accordance with the team spirit which had developed, a farewell meal was arranged for the following month when the new 'house' would have started. Hence, it was one month later that we were all reunited and enjoyed a highly sociable night out. Inevitably, the conversation turned to work within the firm and the consultants reported that things were not going well at all; apparently, there were some problems with the new 'house' ...

Conclusion

This Case Study has described how both the mission goal and the survival task of the firm became threatened. A systems theory analysis might have explained these problems as resulting from an imbalance between the fulfilment of the core task and the mission goal, with the importance of maintaining the research subsystem jeopardising the system itself. However, use of an action approach demonstrated that the differing experiences and expectations of the members influenced the structure and running of the organisation. The juniors' ability to compromise the firm's survival by exercising negative power resulted in a form of negotiated order. In order to explain the needs of the members and the different groups, it was found useful to draw upon neohuman relations theory.

A contingency model of organisation theory offers a means of understanding how future changes of 'house' may affect the unit. The essence of this perspective is the view that the effective operation of an organisation is dependent on there being an appropriate match between its internal organisation and the nature of the demands placed upon it by its tasks, its environment and the needs of its members. The imbalance of these factors in this unit has been described, with some examples of how they affected the organisation. Continued management by the consultants with their interest in research outweighing their clinical commitment, and insensitive personalities without regard for the needs of their junior staff suggests that future 'houses' will affect, and be affected by, the organisation in a similar way to that described. Resolution in this case was wholly dependent on the registrar who was due to leave after one year. Future survival of this unit may well hinge upon whether her successors possess comparable managerial skills.

Case Study 5: Consultants who don't consult

A Senior House Officer

Editors' introduction
The setting for this case study is a general hospital in the period following the Griffiths report. It is noteworthy for the fact that it is an example in which general management has started to get items on the agenda for consultants to consider, albeit in this case a directive from the Department of Health concerning the reduction in junior doctors' hours on call (NHS Management Executive, 1991). As a practical management exercise, it represents the problems of the implementation at local level of a strategy devised nationally but without the addition of earmarked resources.

In spite of this relatively new situation of a willingness of the consultants to respond, apparently without demur, to the request of general management for change, the Case Study illustrates that many traditional values affect the situation. Most of the consultants involved have a belief in the clinical firm, to the extent that they expect the junior doctors attached to their firm to be involved in the firm's admissions, regardless of the unsocial hours. This necessarily leads to a lack of flexibility in rostering on call duties. In addition, there is the hint that the male consultant staff expect a subservient attitude from the predominantly female junior doctors, attitudes which are normally seen more frequently in doctor–nurse relationships.

Organisational perspectives: an action approach (Introduction, pages 28–9) is used to especially good effect in this study to bring out the different motivations and perceptions of the situation of the main groups of doctors involved in the conflict over rotas in the Medical Division. This not only helps to explain the differences of interest which contributed to the emergence of the conflict but also clarified why the consultants were unable to achieve the degree of compliance from their juniors which they seemed to expect.

The Case Study

Some time ago I spent two years working as a Senior House Officer (SHO) in general medicine at a district general hospital in which this account is set. It was a large, relatively modern hospital of some 800 beds and comprised the 'acute' specialties of General Medicine, General Surgery, Obstetrics & Gynaecology, Paediatrics and Psychiatry; as well as wards specialising in rehabilitation and a large Elderly Care Unit with both acute and long-stay beds. The hospital was opened in the 1970s, replacing a nearby smaller unit. Some of the older consultants were originally employed at the old hospital and have had considerable influence over the development of services at the new site.

The General Medical division was made up of the wards and personnel dealing with acute general medical, medical sub-speciality and elderly care patients. This sub-division of the hospital had a total bed complement of around 300 (13 wards); approximately 130 acute general and sub-specialised medical beds as well as 170 elderly care beds. Although the majority of personnel were nurses, paramedical support workers and domestics, they took little or no part in the subsequent events that I wish to describe and full details of their numbers, roles, etc. are not, therefore, given. The division was headed by a 'Clinical Director', one of the consultants chosen by the others to carry the budgetary, administrative and managerial responsibilities of the whole division alongside his own clinical commitment. There was a total of thirty doctors who were considered to constitute the organisation (the Medical Division); of whom twenty junior doctors were at the various grades of senior registrar (SR), registrar (REG), senior house officer (SHO) and house officer (HO).

The organisation, with the exception of the elderly care unit, operated as a collection of 'firms', made up of the individual consultants and their junior staff. Diagram 2.13 shows the hierarchical structure of the medical division and its formation into 'firms'. Diagram 2.14 details the power, roles and responsibilities of the various subgroups.

Each firm had designated wards for patients under the care of each consultant. However, the unpredictable rate of emergency admissions and the varying intensities of different firms' workloads meant that one firm might be responsible for numbers of patients who were distributed on other wards throughout the hospital. These patients were considered to be 'boarding' on another firm's ward so that responsibility for their care rested not with the junior doctors of that ward, but the already overworked juniors whose base ward was elsewhere. Wards were dispersed over a wide area and this could lead to considerable problems for junior staff trying to care for all their patients at once. All juniors rotated to different firms during the course of their job and experienced both very busy and very slack periods.

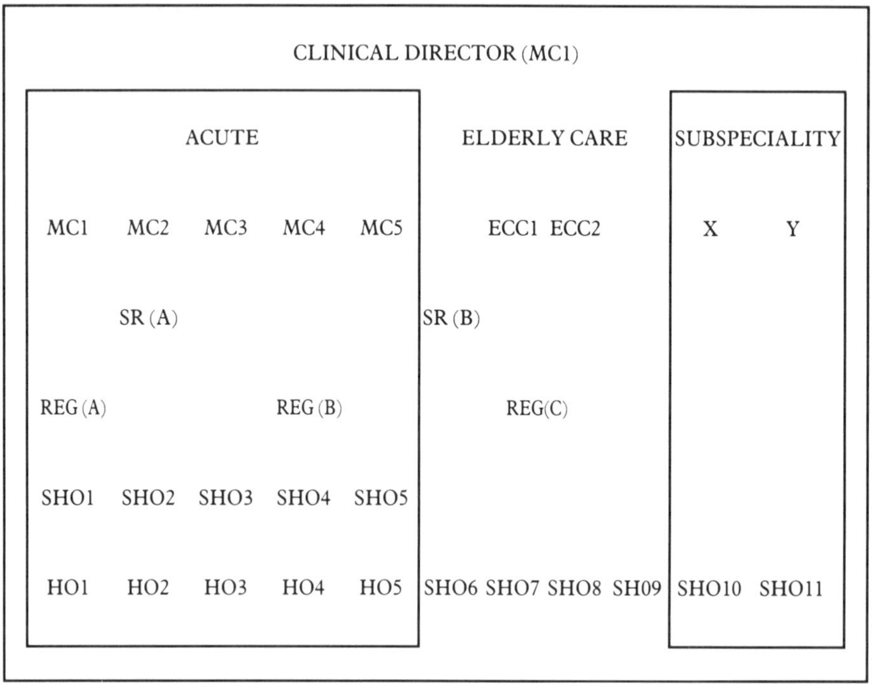

CLINICAL DIRECTOR (MC1)

ACUTE					ELDERLY CARE	SUBSPECIALITY	
MC1	MC2	MC3	MC4	MC5	ECC1 ECC2	X	Y
	SR (A)				SR (B)		
REG (A)			REG (B)		REG(C)		
SHO1	SHO2	SHO3	SHO4	SHO5			
HO1	HO2	HO3	HO4	HO5	SHO6 SHO7 SHO8 SH09	SHO10	SHO11

Diagram 2.13   The formal organisation of Medical Division staff

The night duty and weekend rota

This action analysis, however, primarily deals with the situation which arose regarding night duty rotas. All doctors worked a standard Monday-to-Friday week. Outside these hours, patients were cared for by 'on-call' staff drawn from all the medical firms whose night and week-end work was in addition to their normal forty hour week. The on-call staff formed a reception or 'take' team to deal with emergency patients taken into hospital outside normal working hours and comprising an acute medical consultant (at home but contactable by telephone), the HO and SHO of the same firm and one SR or REG. In addition there was a 'cover' HO or SHO to provide medical care for patients of the other four firms and the sub-specialities.

The planning of night and weekend work involved a complex timetable and to provide the context for this study it is necessary to describe it in some detail. Though the full staff complement at SR/REG level was five, usually only four were in post at the same time. They were permitted to make their own 'on-call' arrangements so that each one worked every fourth night on average, but could choose which night suited them best.

Job title	Role
Consultant	Position of most power and authority within this organisation Responsible for the appropriate treatment of own patients by delegation to juniors Responsible for supervision, training and actions of juniors
Senior Registrar (SR)	Ostensibly a position of some power but: few in number, – belong to neither senior nor junior sub-groups, – close to gaining consultant appointment, thus reluctant to make waves Act as a consultant under supervision and often allowed to decide on therapy Daytime work schedule (clinic sessions, etc.) determined by consultants Construct own night rota (with registrars). Passed postgraduate exams.
Registrar (REG)	Ostensibly a position of some power but again: few in number, – belong to junior sub-groups but want to belong to senior one, – start of career path proper thus both keen to achieve and reluctant to make waves Act under supervision of consultant or SR and occasionally may decide on therapy Daytime work schedule (clinic sessions, etc.) determined by consultants Construct own night rota (with senior registrars). Passed postgraduate exams.
Senior House Officer (SHO)	Minimal power but greatest numbers Act under supervision of the above and provide close check on HO's work Mixed motivations towards role – career/part of other training scheme/job Responsible for smooth running of one consultant's firm, paperwork, etc. Both daytime schedule and night rota imposed by others.
House Officer (HO)	Almost no power Act under supervision of all the above most closely covered by SHOs. Mixed motivations towards role – career/necessary part of gaining full registration Responsible for smooth running of own ward(s), hands-on investigation/treatment of the firm's patients throughout the hospital. Both daytime schedule and night rota imposed by others.

Diagram 2.14   The power, roles and responsibilities of the medical staff

Whilst 'on-call' they had to remain overnight in the hospital mainly in case the SHOs needed advice on the management of the emergency patients being admitted.

One of the consultants had designed a complicated twenty-week cycle rota which ensured that the consultants themselves worked an average of every fifth weekend and every fifth night. Weekend duty was worked as a Friday morning to Saturday lunch time or Saturday morning to Monday teatime shift. SHOs and HOs on-call rotas followed this same pattern so that the SHO and HO of one firm would be on-call together when 'taking' emergency patients. Each would also work every twentieth night as 'cover'. The four SHOs attached to the elderly care department worked an average of every fourth night and weekend providing cover for patients on the elderly care unit. Thus each SHO and HO worked every fourth night overall, though this might mean working four nights one week and only one the next.

It was the consultants' view that continuity of care, the patient being admitted by the junior members of one consultant's firm, was of paramount importance and once secured all other considerations were unimportant. However, this 'rule' did not seem to apply when consultants went on leave. Duties were readily swapped with another consultant in the knowledge that he or she was likely to remain undisturbed at home for most of their on-call. All-in-all, the rota was immensely complex, worked out months in advance but did not allow for junior staff taking annual study or sick leave. If they had to be away for any of these reasons the system crashed. An example of the rota is shown below in Diagram 2.15.

	Mon	Tues	Wed	Thurs	Fri	Sat/Sun
Week 1	Take		Cover			Take
Week 2		Take				
Week 3					Take	
Week 4	Cover			Take		
Week 5			Take			

Diagram 2.15   Junior doctors' night and weekend roster

This rota ran for some time during which there was increasing dissatisfaction amongst the junior doctors who had to operate it. Eventually, attempts to change the system triggered open conflict between the consultants and the SHOs and HOs. To place this confrontation in context and explain how it developed, it is first necessary to describe the main actors in the drama and to seek to define their involvement with the organisation. A helpful method of approach to this is to use an action perspective and to consider in turn the goals and motivation of the main groups of professionals within the Division and try to construct a picture of how each group saw its situation within the organisation.

The actors

All members of the organisation probably shared the formal goal: to provide the best possible treatment for all patients referred to the hospital with medical disorders. Beyond this, the threat of legal action by a patient, or proposed cutbacks in funding from the regional or district health authorities also produced a 'united front' response. After this point, however, perspectives were likely to differ. Only the *consultant* group were likely to own secondary aims which included the survival and expansion of the medical division within the hospital, and the survival of the hospital *per se*, as this group alone were contracted to the hospital for more than the next two years. The *SR*s, *REG*s, *SHO*s and *HO*s aimed to impress their seniors, on whom they relied for a reference to help them secure their next job. This was even more important for the SRs and REGs who also need a degree of patronage to help them succeed in their chosen field. For all juniors the unspoken threat that failure to play by the rules of the organisation may be rewarded by a poor reference is a real one, and acts to maintain the *status quo*.

Another explicit aim of the organisation was, in theory at least, the training and education of junior doctors. However, the consultants showed variable evidence of commitment to this in their dealings with SHOs and HOs, and their available teaching time was most often taken up by undergraduate medical students, SRs and REGs. Given the constraints imposed by the hours of work, there was little opportunity for SHOs and HOs to study outside duty hours. It was hardly surprising, then, that SHOs and HOs were likely to perceive the organisation as an entity whose main purpose was to prevent them from sleeping at night. Using these various perceptions it is possible to construct 'Ideal Types', that is the characteristics typifying the various roles. *Consultants* were responsible for the care of patients referred to them and for the training and education of their juniors. They were also responsible for the development of their own fields of interest such as research, equipment, staffing levels, and out-patient clinics. *Registrar and Senior Registrar* grade staff took responsibility for ensuring that consultants' instructions for patient care were carried out by the SHOs and HOs and for undertaking all the tasks a consultant felt were beneath him or that were more appropriate for them. They also needed to be seen to help develop the division or the field of interest to ensure a good reference and so further their own career. Although technically part of the junior staff, their motivations were so different that I have considered them separately from the SHOs and HOs.

The SHOs and HOs taken together, form what I will refer to as the 'juniors'. They had to carry out routine treatment and investigation of patients as instructed, and decide on the appropriate investigations and treatment for emergency patients. In short they were expected to ensure that emergency patients lived to see the consultant next day. This group was also responsible for interviewing and examining all patients, organising notes and results, prescribing drugs and intravenous fluids, inserting intravenous cannulae, booking tests, administering most injections, writing discharge summaries and any job too mundane or unpleasant to be done by other staff. One of their main goals was to avoid being shouted at.

Turning now to look more specifically at the motivation of these different groups, the consultant staff seemed to have a predominantly moral motivation which was demonstrated by their commitment to the well-being of the individual patient, to the hospital, to their own department and the existence of their own firm of junior staff. The clinical director, *MC 1*, shared this moral motivation which also encompassed his role as budget holder for the division. He was, therefore, motivated to ensure everyone stayed within budget and so needed power, authority and legitimacy. He had a personal desire for order and routine and intense commitment to his own career to the point of being seen as a 'workaholic'. Unfortunately this seemed to restrict his ability to comprehend or appreciate juniors who were less committed. He showed evidence of alienative motivation in his personal antipathy towards *MC 5* and the desire to be seen to 'score points' at the other's expense. Consultant *MC 3* shared the moral motivation of his peer group but also had affective motivation in that he seemed to have a strong personal need to be liked and appreciated. It is also relevant for this case study to record that he owned a computer on which he was keen to demonstrate his expertise. Consultant *MC 5* was the only remaining acute medical consultant who had initially practised at the old hospital. He had previously been the clinical director and was responsible for increasing the levels of staff, equipment and prestige over time and was well respected by other consultants. Again he shared the moral motivation of his colleagues to his work but also demonstrated alienative motivation in his strong antipathy towards one of them, *MC 1*, based on his views of the latter's medical judgement, administrative capacity and personnel management abilities. Nevertheless, he wanted to be seen to rise above *MC 1*'s jibes and also showed personal commitment to the juniors in his own firm, as well as genuine concern at the level of unhappiness demonstrated by the majority of the SHOs and HOs.

All junior staff showed moral motivation by their commitment to the individual patient. Registrars were also motivated in an instrumental fashion by the need to 'win friends' to further their own career progression and the avoidance of any situations, such as disagreement over hours of work, which might lead to them being seen as not 100 per cent committed to their chosen specialty. As a group, the SHOs and HOs seemed to be motivated by a mixture of factors. There were clearly affective elements in their commitment to an individual consultant and strong ties to others in their own grade, the 'fellow sufferers'. They also exhibited alienative elements due to the lack of commitment to the hospital, the lack of commitment to their own department (as they rotated on a four-monthly basis throughout the division) and the fact that their career plan might not be to become a general medical consultant. They also seemed to be motivated by purely instrumental elements. These could include such factors as perceiving the current post as a means to an end, ie it would enable them to enter, or continue along, their chosen career path, as for example to become a general practitioner.

SHO 1 and *SHO 4* shared the moral motivation of this group. They also had strong affective motivation in their close personal friendship with each other and in their good relationships with various consultants, due in part to the fact that they were the longest serving junior members of staff at that time. However, there were limits to their motivation to the hospital in general and their firms within it in particular, as both had chosen careers outside general medicine and had already secured new posts. This also meant, of course, that neither was likely to be influenced by the threat of a poor reference. Both were newly married, and unsurprisingly, were also motivated by a desire to spend time with their new partners.

The action analysis of these different subgroups is summarised in Diagram 2.16.

Proposals for a new deal and their rejection

After many months of informal comments from the SHOs and HOs about the unsuitability of the rota, the Department of Health, responding to national debate on the issue of junior doctors' hours, proposed its 'New Deal' limiting the maximum period these doctors could work in any one week and began to apply pressure at general management level for its implementation. This meant that in our hospital the general manager started to ask all hospital consultants about their juniors' hours and the issue was suddenly on the agenda.

SHO 1 was unexpectedly accosted by *MC 3*. He explained that both he and *MC 1* were aware there were problems with the rota, and they were keen to improve the situation. This came as no little surprise to the SHO who was more used to hearing these two consultants express the opinion that in comparison to how hard they had had to work, today's juniors didn't know when they were well off. She immediately offered help in

Categories	Main motivation/commitment				Definition of situation	Actions taken
	Moral	Affect-ive	Instru-mental	Alien-ative		
Consultants	+				**Favourable/Mixed:** External pressure to change 'We did it and it didn't hurt us', Wary that juniors' conditions would improve at own expense	**Passive** response Delegated responsibility to the Clinical Director. He then formed a horizontal clique with a second consultant, who had a computer
SRs and Registrars	+		+		**Favourable/Mixed:** 'We did it etc . . .', Wary that improvement for SHOs/HOs would be at own expense. Had worked in worse places to advance own career	**Passive** response initially. Later tried to convince SHOs and HOs that since other places were worse, they should accept their lot
SHOs and HOs	+			+	**Unfavourable:** All aspects – hours of duty, actual tasks inappropriate, inflexible rota, lack of consultation	**Passive** Circumvention of rota and certain tasks to point of active resistance **Active** response later, using threats of non-co-operation
MC1 and MC3	+				**Favourable (Mixed):** Aware that rota worse in other places	**Active** response, designed new rotas without consultation. Vertical clique with SHO 1
MC5	+	+			**Unfavourable**	**Active** response, Supportive of HOs and SHOs in background, Devil's advocate, Vertical clique with SHO 4
SHO1 and SHO4	+	+		+	**Unfavourable**	**Active** part in cliques as above. Information exchange among SHOs/HOs. Formal and informal negotiation within and between sub-groups

Diagram 2.16 An action analysis of relationships in the Medical Division

pointing out areas of greatest concern to the junior staff, but was rebuffed. The two consultants proposed altering the current system whereby juniors worked all or part of every alternate weekend (as previously explained) to decrease continuous hours of duty. This would require them to work a smaller part of three weekends in every four. They also planned to devise a new 'computer' rota for all night duty. She tried to suggest that working almost every weekend, whether it reduced overall hours or not, was highly unlikely to appeal to the juniors. In her view the best way to achieve a reduction in hours satisfactory to all groups would be to involve representatives of the juniors in any discussions. However, she was promptly informed by the two consultants that she didn't understand the situation. *SHO 1* decided to discuss these events with the other juniors.

There was evidently a great difference in the way that the various groups perceived the situation. Consultants 1 and 3 showed little genuine concern for the juniors' conditions and seemed preoccupied with appeasing management and the Department of Health. They did not feel that the consultation or participation of the group most directly affected was in any way necessary. The sixteen juniors met informally. They quickly realised that since the rota needed four people to be present at night, and a weekend comprised three nights, they would have very few free weekends even if no-one took annual leave. There was no support for a reduction in hours by these means, which was seen to be worse than the present system. The juniors asked *SHO 1* to arrange a formal meeting with the two consultants. This took place shortly afterwards between all the juniors and *MC1*, as head of division. Despite their hopes that this might mark the start of two-way consultation or negotiation, *MC 1* simply expressed extreme disappointment that the juniors were not prepared to use this opportunity to reduce their hours. His attempts at applying emotional blackmail were not successful. He did not seem to appreciate that to persuade someone to accept a change in the *status quo* to their own detriment, solely to please the person requesting the change, requires there to be an affective motivation towards that individual. The juniors were well aware of the external pressures on *MC 1* to be seen to have made progress in this field. Since the possibility of negotiation was denied to them, they chose the only course they could see which allowed them to gain some power. They informed *MC 1* that he could introduce a new rota but it would not be utilised. Since they were also aware that a material change to a contract of employment requires the consent of both parties, they felt on reasonably safe ground. The meeting finished.

The consultants' second attempt: a trial scheme

After a lull of a couple of weeks, *SHO 1* was again approached by *MC 3*. She was given a new rota and asked if she would canvass the opinions of one or two of the SHOs. She was given the impression that it would be appreciated if she would only discuss it with SHOs who were likely to look favourably on it, and that it would be best if this rota was accepted since it did not involve dividing up the weekends. This new development was informally discussed by the SHOs and HOs. It did contain some improvements. Rather than increased numbers of staff working at weekends, those working would exchange duties on Sunday, thereby evening out the different intensities of the various jobs. However, there were some major drawbacks. This new rota involved the creation of a sixth emergency admittance team, using the SHOs from elderly care and the subspecialties who would also have to cope with their routine workloads. Since the elderly care department was separate from the medical wards, this would entail considerable disruption in the daily work pattern of some SHOs, and would mean that often only three SHOs would be available to cope with a workload previously carried by four. Nonetheless, night duties would be more evenly spread across all personnel, who would admit emergencies every sixth night and provide internal medical cover every twelfth night. The SRs and registrars advised the SHOs to accept the new rota and stop rocking the boat.

After discussion, the HOs and SHOs felt that the rota was far from ideal as it did not reduce overall hours and a small number of SHOs would carry increased duties for the same wage. However, it seemed to be the best on offer in a situation where formal negotiation was not a possibility. The SHOs, therefore, agreed to accept the new rota but only on a trial basis. *SHO 4* was then quietly approached by *MC 5*, expressing his disquiet at the railroading of the junior staff into unacceptable rotas and his desire to help. Informal discussions were instituted by the SHO, centring on the removal of the 'firm' system of working. Though *MC 5* was not at all keen on the idea of relinquishing this system, he accepted that there was no way that a real change in hours could be achieved without creating a new more flexible pattern of working. His aims in offering help and support appeared two-fold. He had a genuine concern to see improvement, led by those on the ground who actually had to work the system, but was also strongly motivated by the desire to succeed where his rival was struggling. He agreed to speak to the other consultants about altering the 'firm' system to a more flexible pattern of work.

Failure and confrontation

In the meantime, the new rota came into operation. It quickly became evident that although the division of roles within a weekend period of duty was beneficial to most, the SHOs in the subspecialties and elderly care were hard pressed to cope with the changes in their daily work patterns. An increasing proportion of their time was spent walking between widely separated wards and answering 'bleeps' from irate nurses, who despite repeated explanations from the SHOs could not comprehend that though an SHO might not be on a certain ward, this did not imply that the SHO had nothing to do. Patient care and the morale of doctors and nurses was suffering. After a two month trial period, the SHOs arranged a further meeting with *MC 1*. They explained that with the best will in the world, the new system was not workable. His response was that they were deliberately trying to sabotage his plans and that they would just have to make the best of it. The SHOs who were directly affected by this were offended both by the inference of intentional disruption and his refusal to honour the arrangements for a trial period. Having been denied any input in planning their own working arrangements, and not being permitted to negotiate, they took 'evasive action'. Of the total eleven SHOs, four immediately went on sick leave. The elderly care and subspecialty consultants were not best pleased at the sudden disappearance of their SHOs, especially since they had less recourse to SRs and REGs than *MC 1*.

SHO 4 discussed these new developments with *MC 5*. *MC 5*, in turn, then spoke to all the other consultants and also told *MC 1* exactly what he thought of his abilities in the field of personnel management. The relationship between these two was deteriorating rapidly, to the extent that *MC 1* found it necessary to make disparaging comments about *MC 5* at a meeting attended by the whole medical division, as well as other hospital staff. This did not improve *MC 1*'s standing, but marked him out as behaving rather childishly and resorting to rudeness when thwarted. The consultants as a group announced that a further review of the rota would commence, remaining under the scrutiny of *MC 1* and *MC 3*. However, this again took place without any formal consultation with or representation of SHOs or HOs. The consultant body asked *REG (A)* to act as the sole junior representative in the discussions. Needless to say *REG (A)*, being closer to the top of the clinical hierarchy than the SHOs and HOs, held views much closer to those of the consultants, and agreed their proposals for the implementation of a new rota after minimal discussion with his junior colleagues. The rota was again devised on *MC 3*'s computer and had similar faults to the other rotas already described. The new scheme would involve doing away with the recently created sixth emergency admittance team, and starting to take more patients directly to the elderly care department. The responsibility for providing cover for patients already in hospital would now fall on the SHO and HO who were admitting emergency patients, thus reducing the 'on-call' team to three. To hopefully spread the workload more evenly, elderly emergency admissions would now be seen by the doctor on call for the elderly care department, rather than those responsible for acute admissions.

There was a final meeting of *MC 1*, *REG (A)* and *SHOs 1* and *4*. By this stage, the SHOs' and HOs' contracts were within a week or two of expiry, and they all had new posts organised, which made them somewhat blasé. *MC 1* made it clear he considered that the current eleven SHOs, who had been predominately female, had been a particularly obstructive group. With the end of the 'house' they were soon to be replaced by a new group, which had deliberately chosen to be dissimilar. He obviously felt that with the departure of the difficult juniors and their replacement with a more reasonable group, the rota problems would sort themselves out. The two SHOs were unimpressed and pointed out that the new system, which was asking three people to take responsibility for up to 300 patients at once, was cutting into safety margins. They also reminded the consultant that the incoming group of SHOs had signed contracts when the original rota was still in operation, so a material change in their working conditions would require their consent. Furthermore, they told *MC 1* that they were aware that reducing the on-call team to three people would save approximately £14,000 to £16,000 a year from the divisional budget; and that since juniors were to be asked to do the same amount of work for less pay this money should be used to provide ancillary staff to assist in the juniors' duties. *MC 1* was not impressed at all by this but agreed to discuss it with the other consultants.

A final meeting of the consultant body was then held at which *MC 5* convinced the other consultants that this money should be used to institute a service for the taking of routine blood samples by technical staff. Furthermore, the consultants agreed to undertake discussions with senior nurses to see if more of the routine ward-based work could be undertaken by them. Unfortunately, he was not able to secure their agreement to include SHO and HO representatives in any future discussions about their own conditions of work.

Outcome

Although the immediate situation was resolved to a certain level of satisfaction to all interested parties, the situation remained one of continuing conflict and flux. The consultants, especially *MC 1*, generally felt that the new intake might well be more malleable, partly as they were predominantly male, in contrast to our mainly female 'house' which had given them so much trouble. They also felt that the revised situation was a favourable one. However, they were facing an unknown quantity who were themselves well aware of the previous situation.

The SRs and REGs were staying in post. They were confident that the new staff would take to the new rota and things could return to normal. They felt that the revised situation was a favourable one. The SHOs, who were all leaving, were relieved that they would not have to continue in this situation. However, *SHOs 1* and *4* were very aware that negotiation had never really been entered into, so no power had been given up by the consultants. Since no other mechanism had been devised in place of negotiation, future problems would likely provoke the same response of threat and counter-threat. Though some concessions had been gained the underlying situation was unchanged. The potential for further conflict remained and continued to undermine the good relationships between the consultants and junior doctors.

After this case study was written, I returned to the hospital to find out what has happened subsequently. The junior staff were still awaiting the appointment of a technician for taking routine blood samples, although a Saturday morning ECG service has been provided. The revised rota arrangements were even less satisfactory than those they replaced. The new, mainly male, SHO intake have not transpired to be the paragons of virtue that some of the consultants were expecting. A registrar resigned and, in the absence of a suitable replacement, one of the SHOs has been asked to fill the position in an unofficial capacity. Another SHO left at short notice and was replaced by someone whose skills were insufficient for the needs of the post. The problems resulting from this staffing shortfall, as juniors' responsibilities have been redefined to cover the necessary work, have allowed morale to fall to an all time low. Despite this, there has been still no agreement by the consultant body to involve the junior staff in determining their own 'on-call' rotas, and the firm system persists. It was a not unexpected continuation of events but it remains difficult to see how it could be altered so long as consultants, who hold so much power and authority in such situations, so strongly resist any change.

Case Study 6: The death of the unicorn and the birth of the Shetland pony: Conflict between Consultants in a Paediatric Unit

A Senior House Officer

Editors' introduction

It is interesting that the style of working of the consultants with their colleagues in this Case Study is similar to their clinical approach to patients. It is often said that good management involves the use of differing styles at different times to cope with diverse kinds of problems. This does not appear to be the situation in this Case Study, since there is an apparent consistency of approach by each consultant (*Consultant A* being consistently inconsistent) and probably accounts for the coalitions that develop around them. Nevertheless, *Consultant B* uses techniques which endear her to general management, for example through the use of efficient measures to provide information quickly in computerised form. Variations of this form of playing the management game will probably become increasingly important for consultants in the future as they find ways to meet the targets, contracts and performance indicators which form the management culture of the new NHS.

Organisational perspectives: the main emphasis in the analysis in this Case Study relies on an action approach (Introduction, pages 28–9), which is used to show the different work and leadership styles of the two consultants who are its principal subject, and to explore the changing pattern of relationships and power which emerge in consequence of these differences. Subsequently, the perspectives of systems, bureaucracy, and human relations (Introduction, pages 22–7) are drawn on to show how a number of factors came together to drain power away from one consultant and draw it into a new dominant coalition led by the other. This study illustrates very clearly the value of being able to take a long view of the history of an organisation such as this in coming to a meaningful interpretation of its contemporary power structure.

The Case Study

Introduction

The aim of this Case Study is to show how the locus of power in a health organisation can shift without any planning or formal intervention by management, and to consider some of the consequences of such a change for those involved. The study falls into three main sections: the first establishes the context, the second examines the evolution of power within the unit concerned, and the third considers the impact of the changes on staff and patients involved.

The information was collected by participant observation, largely by myself but the observations of others were included. Rudimentary analysis commenced while I was working in the unit but the more detailed and considered evaluation of the case was carried out after I had moved on to my next job and was assisted by further contact with other people still working in the unit for updates on subsequent developments. The main advantage of participant observations is access afforded to the hidden agenda. This has three particular elements: (1) appreciation of the operational structure and goals of the organisation and the individuals in it; (2) eye witness accounts of relationships, conflicts and alliances of power; (3) receipt of the confidences of members of key interest groups. Taken together, these facilitate the gathering of what might be termed 'experimental evidence'.

It is difficult to refute allegations that work of this type is prone to subjectivity and memory bias. This study is not, however, a randomised control trial of differing organisational types. It is a descriptive work, the very worth of which is in its subjectivity as it allows recognition by readers of the similarities within their own organisation. To critics, it should be said that this tool of participant observation, whilst it is difficult to validate the findings formally, is the means by which many expositions of organisational theory are made in the expert literature. The memory bias factor may also be largely discounted as this work was first drafted less than nine months after the observation period ended.

To the writer, the success of this study will be measured by the receipt of vision and empowerment by those who have previously been pawns in similar situations.

My involvement in the paediatric unit was as an SHO on a six month attachment as part of a rotation in the medical specialities. My duties involved the out-patient care of children with chronic diseases, including that medical and social involvement usually reserved for the primary health care team. Informal out-patient assessments were carried out in the ward area and I was also required to assist at formal out-patient clinics. I was also responsible for the 14 bed ward, caring for in-patients with acute exacerbations or complications of their condition as well as those with incidental illnesses. Care was also provided to children having surgery. I took part in the Special Care Baby Unit/Intensive Care Unit rota, caring for babies with problems associated with prematurity, nutritional problems, cardiac, respiratory or renal failure. I was resident on call every third night and third weekend, and shared this rota with two registrars.

I have not considered my own involvement in the case study as it was of marginal importance and confined to only six months in a development which spanned several years.

The history of the unit

The Paediatric Unit is in a large general hospital, next to a University. It was established in the early 1970s as a satellite of the main Regional unit in the hospital adjoining the medical school. The original aim of the satellite unit was to provide basic first line care for local children with certain chronic diseases. It is now one of a growing number of units in the Region as specialisation increases with technological advance. The catchment population is estimated at 1,000,000. The unit provides specialist secondary and tertiary services to several District Health Authorities. It is in the process of establishing itself as part of a trust. The facilities for which the unit is equipped have also expanded, now providing complete care of patients requiring acute, chronic or intensive care. A few very specialised interventions are still only provided in the Regional Centre.

Initially the unit was founded by a general paediatrician. He was an enthusiast, largely self taught, and an elder statesman figure. Subsequently, it was championed by a younger paediatrician, *Consultant A*, who had some training in the care of children with certain chronic diseases. His training took place outside the Region. He was appointed around the time that the unit opened. The second consultant, *Consultant B*, was appointed several years later in the early 1980s. She was also a specialist, having trained in the Regional Unit. Since she took up her post, the number of patients requiring the unit's specialist expertise has approximately doubled.

Formal Structure

Function of the organisation
I have chosen to study the function of the organisation by viewing it as an open system that aimed at achieving equilibrium by the adoption and success of primary and mission tasks. Analysis by this method enables one to see the rise of the dominant coalition as the triumph of the task over the taskmaster.

Unit tasks
The primary task of any organisation is survival. The unit will survive for as long as it can provide specialist facilities for the local population cheaper than with unit closure. The mission tasks of an organisation (or unit within an organisation) can be regarded as those tasks pursued by the controlling members of the enterprise which are over and above the tasks which must be fulfilled for its survival. In the Paediatric Unit it was possible to identify three such goals:

1. Expansion of the facility such that all patients who are eligible can be offered the most appropriate form of specialist care, eg by expansion of the services to cover the early and late evening and early mornings.
2. Improvement in the quality of life of the patients. (a) By the purchase of new equipment, allowing interventions to be more closely tailored to patient requirements thus reducing the side effects of treatment. (b) By progressive therapy. Patients with certain chronic conditions are prone to disabling complications. This unit aims to minimise both the incidence and the effects of these by monitoring blood levels and emphasising prevention and early treatment.
3. Avoidance of crisis. When the condition of a child deteriorates it may

do so very rapidly and with serious consequences. An open access system, enabling patients to telephone the unit to arrange urgent assessment or admission was considered important as planned management was seen as far more satisfactory than constant crisis.

To achieve these tasks the Paediatric Unit was divided into a formal structure of two main sections: the In-Patient Unit and the Specialist Out-Patient Unit. The main roles and responsibilities in the Paediatric Unit are summarised in Diagram 2.17, below.

Consultant
Overall clinical management
Co-ordination of short/long-term goals
Care of acute and chronic patients

Medical Unit Nurse Manager
Overall co-ordination of nursing service,
reduction of conflict.

Dietician
Provision of professional dietary advice to
medical and nursing staff.
Interception of unsuitable foods from hospital kitchen.

In-Patient Unit	Specialist Out-Patient Unit
SISTER	SISTER/CHARGE NURSE
Co-ordination and	Co-ordination and management
management of acutely	of specialist nursing
ill patients.	of ITU patients.
Recovery from interventions.	Assessment of patients.
Stabilisation on ongoing	Pre- and post-intervention
treatment.	monitoring health status and
	levels of disease activity.

Staff/Enrolled Nurse
First line care of all patients.
Drug administration.

Technicians
Care and maintenance of machinery.

Diagram 2.17 The main roles and responsibilities in the Paediatric Unit

The power structure within the organisation

The two Consultants

It is often assumed by those who write as independent observers of different sections or units of the NHS that the source of all professional power lies with doctors. Whilst this is shown to be only partly true in this study, it is a logical place to begin the study of power in the Paediatric Unit.

The two consultants working in the Unit will be referred to throughout as *Consultant A* and *Consultant B*. *Consultant A* was male, and active in pursuit of personal outside interests, whereas *Consultant B* was female, and active within the community. They were of opposing political persuasions. In certain parts of the country the Paediatric Unit was known as '*Consultant A*'s Unit' whilst in others it was '*Consultant B*'s Unit'. The power situation which I discovered when I began my six months with the organisation had changed quite dramatically over the years since *Consultant B* was recruited to join *Consultant A* in running the Unit. Prior to that time *Consultant A* had been in sole clinical command of all the unit's activities. From discussion with other staff who had stayed with the unit since that era, it was possible to put together a picture of the distribution of power and authority that prevailed then, and to establish a good idea of the processes which had led to the subsequent changes.

Consultant A in the ascendancy:
the dominant coalition in the early 1980s
When *Consultant B* first joined the unit to take over responsibility for the Specialist Out-patient Clinic, all the evidence suggests that *Consultant A* was regarded as the unchallenged leader of the whole unit. Although after *Consultant B* was appointed, the two consultants took lead responsibility for different clinical areas which *Consultant A* had previously held. He remained secure in the allegiance of all the senior nursing and technical staff whether they were in his clinical area or *Consultant B*'s. The impetus built up by several years of his strong, charismatic leadership lasted well into the new regime of shared clinical command. The dominant coalition of the time is represented in Diagram 2.18.

Consultant A★	**Consultant B**
In-patient Unit	*Specialist Out-patient Unit*
Sister P★	Charge Nurse F★
Staff Nurse A★	Sister A★
	Staff Nurse K★
	Technician C★

★ = member of the dominant coalition

Diagram 2.18   The dominant coalition in the Paediatric Unit
in the early 1980s

The evolution of power relationships in the Unit: seven years later
Nevertheless, by the time of my arrival in the Unit seven years after *Consultant B*, a new set of power relationships prevailed. In terms of work responsibilities a more equal position appeared to exist. However, in other respects it seemed that the dominance of *Consultant A* continued, at least in terms of his image and personal perks. Closer acquaintance with the

Unit, however, showed that these perceptions of the consultants' positions were unreliable as indicators of the real distribution of power in the Unit and it became clear that a radical realignment had taken place leading to the emergence of a new dominant coalition led by *Consultant B*.

Clinical duties
During my time in the Unit, there were five specialist clinics each week. Four of these were undertaken by *Consultant B* and one was shared. Both consultants attended the twice weekly in-patient ward round and a 1 in 2 on call rota was on a 'week about' basis. The consultants also shared a general paediatric workload, including responsibility for patients requiring special or intensive care. *Consultant A* did the larger part of this work, balancing the greater involvement of *Consultant B* in specialist out-patient care. Their peak activity times during the day were also different. *Consultant A* was a morning person who often arrived on the unit before the first group of patients and dealt with a.m. crises. *Consultant B* arrived later but often worked late into the evening and was the person of choice for afternoon/evening crises.

This situation would appear to have allowed a more equitable power sharing arrangement than most. The number of hours during which the consultants were available on the unit was certainly greater than in other similar situations. However, there were other minor but possibly significant indications suggesting that *Consultant A* continued to be in the stronger position of the two.

There had been a complaint that one of the consultants was inaccessible, but which one? *Consultant A* was often absent pursuing his outside, vaguely medically related interests. These occasionally required him to be away from the Unit at short notice. He also dabbled in private practice, and his other hobbies sometimes found him difficult to obtain. *Consultant B*'s absences, however, were more easily justifiable in the pursuit of health goals. She religiously attended postgraduate meetings, spent much time planning the service and fighting for more resources. She also sat on local council committees and frequently took up and won her patients' battles for employment, housing and suchlike.

Interestingly, the complaint that was made was against *Consultant B* as she was frequently late for morning clinics, whereas *Consultant A* was always early.

The room with a view: the perks of power?
The hospital has a small postgraduate centre which includes a largely donated library, a seminar room and the offices of most consultants and their secretaries. *Consultant A*'s office was in this centre. It was small but modern and well furnished. The view, whilst not picturesque, was at least of the outside world and the windows opened when required. *Consultant*

B's office, in contrast, was on a corridor separate from the others. It was slightly larger but less accessible. The furnishings were older and shabbier, the window was barred and the view was of a lift shaft. It was a dull, dingy and depressing place. This cursory examination suggests that *Consultant A*, having been established longer, being more prominent in public relations, having the better office and superficially the greater support of the patients, was the more powerful actor. That was my opinion when I took up my position but I soon learned how ill-founded it was.

The distribution of power and authority within the organisation

Diagram 2.19 opposite outlines the networks of power within the Unit as I came to perceive them during my time there. There were two main interest groups, the first led by *Consultant A* and associated with the in-patient unit: the second by *Consultant B* and identified with the specialist out-patient unit. *Consultant A* remained a charismatic figure. Multi-talented and superior, he enjoyed reigning over those who expected and, in their turn, sought to impose a hierarchical structure. *Consultant B* was hardly charismatic but was a professional beaver, expert, consistent and egalitarian. It was the interest group involving *Consultant B* which was in the ascendancy and could be considered the dominant coalition.

The dominant coalition

Diagram 2.20 below is a simplified version of Diagram 2.19 showing only the main actors. That is not to say that those omitted had neither power nor allegiance, merely that they were decision influencers rather than decision directors.

Consultant A	**Consultant B★**
In-patient Unit	*Specialist Out-patient Unit*
Sister P	Charge Nurse F@ Sister A Sister B
Staff Nurse A@	Staff Nurse B@ Staff Nurse K@
Enrolled Nurse I@	
	Technician I@
	Technician C
★ Dominant Coalition	

Diagram 2.20 Membership of the dominant coalition in the
Paediatric Unit in the late 1980s

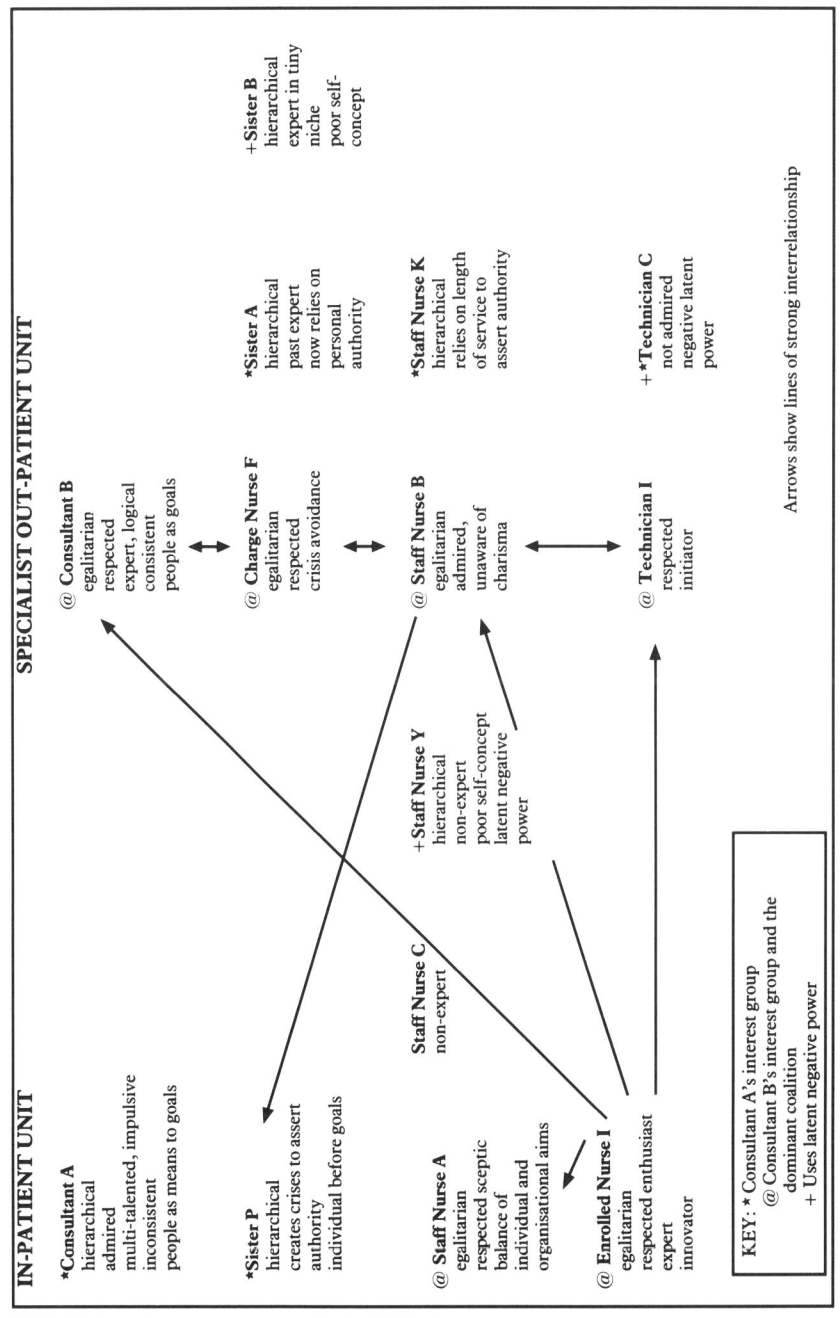

Diagram 2.19 Power, authority and commitment in the
Paediatric Unit in the late 1980s

It became clear that a polar situation had developed between the two interest groups for three main reasons:

1. Survival of the Specialist Unit. The members of the dominant coalition were committed to the continued growth and success of the Unit. Unlike *Consultant A*, the former leader of the dominant coalition, their energies were not diluted by activities elsewhere.

2. Distance between the In-patient Unit and the Specialist Out-patient Unit. The In-patient Unit was situated some distance from the Specialist Out-patient Unit. In the former, the fabric was in poor condition whilst the latter was specially built. The units were staffed independently, neither numbers nor skill mix were coordinated. This resulted not only in isolation of the two units but staff shortages on the In-patient Unit had led to friction as Specialist Out-patient Unit staff had been required to help on the ward. This, particularly through the strength of the influence of *Enrolled Nurse I*, a highly energetic and effective 'lower participant' and strong advocate of *Consultant B*, had reinforced the general dominance of the Specialist Out-patient Unit.

3. Distribution of expertise. Specialist Unit staff carried out technical interventions, assessed and taught patients how to monitor their disease. They also carried out some technical interventions in the intensive care unit and assisted in minor specialist surgical procedures undertaken in the unit. Some specialist interventions were also undertaken by in-patient staff. These were, however, less technical procedures which were mostly carried out on older children whose disease was less severe. For these reasons such procedures were considered less demanding.

Admitting patients for such interventions was also expensive. The number of such procedures was gradually being reduced, for as more gentle methods of intervention developed and side effects lessened, so the indications for undertaking different procedures in children with less severe symptoms diminished.

Specialist Unit staff were thus seen as more talented. This view was reinforced by the nursing hierarchy who allowed Specialist Unit staff more clinical freedom and responsibility, eg the taking of blood samples and administration of intravenous drugs.

Understanding the ascendancy of the new dominant coalition

As the diagram of the key actors illustrates, the interest group led by *Consultant B* had become the dominant coalition. This had largely been the triumph of the expert over the charismatic. The power of the charismatic can be seen to have declined for several reasons. An analysis of the organisation from various perspectives can help to establish a broad understanding of how this came about.

Considering the organisation as a system

Whilst a charismatic leader is often the prime mover behind the founding of an organisation, as it develops, his or her global enthusiasm for all its goals can wane and be replaced by a narrower commitment to a mission task at the expense of the primary task. In this organisation, where survival depended on satisfying several complex criteria, a key figure dedicated to the survival of the unit was obviously essential. The main interest of *Consultant A* was in the second mission task: improvement in quality of life. His energy, however, was devoted to a small subgroup of patients only, those requiring intensive care. It can be seen, therefore, that *Consultant B*, with her work on resources and important academic contacts, became also the systems maintenance engineer.

Professional bureaucracy

The NHS is frequently seen as a professional bureaucracy. It is true that appointment is largely by demonstrated competence. There are written codes of conduct, and maintenance of order is necessary to ensure a degree of standardisation and universality of coverage. In the main, consultants use the bureaucratic machinery to serve their own organisation. *Consultant B* did this by her insistence on setting up computerised information systems enabling essential written communications to be handled speedily. This in turn improved the Unit's status with the holders of the purse strings in the NHS bureaucracy of which it was a part.

Consultant A, however, was an advocate of adhocracy, of the expensive, the eccentric and the esoteric whether in the predictable daily round or in crisis. This approach had the potential to jeopardise the greater good of the routine majority who required the machinery of the professional bureaucracy to ensure the smooth delivery of service.

Human relations model

It has been argued that the network of influence related to charismatic leaders allows more scope for personal creativity and the attainment of higher levels of self-actualisation within an organisation. In the In-patient Unit, however, this was far from clear. The unpredictable treatment plans of the consultant and his authoritarian style of management left the sceptics asking 'What does my creativity create? What is the impact of my self-actualisation beyond my own development?'. It seemed in practice that there was much greater self actualisation amongst the more egalitarian group of staff led by *Consultant B* who felt they had a measure of control over both their own and the organisation's destinies.

The leadership of *Consultant A* was really a modern variant of that imposed by a McGregor's *Theory X* leader (McGregor, 1960) masquerading as a human relations practitioner, meeting some higher needs but in reality providing for little basic self-determination. The concept of alignment is helpful in illuminating the consequences of the situation. Alignment here is taken to mean the matching of personal values, skills and interests with the task requirements of the job, resulting in an orientation that maximises both the fulfilment of the needs of the individual and the organisation. The promotion of alignment is obviously a means of achieving both stability and high output in an organisation of professionals like the Specialist Out-patient Unit. Where, as was apparently the case in the Unit at the time, the dominant coalition has identified its own interests with those of the organisation; this may become a self perpetuating situation. In contrast, in the In-patient Unit the evidence for alignment of individual and organisational needs was much less evident.

Political model
The progressive reduction of alignment amongst the members of the charismatic leader's team can also be seen as involving the gradual erosion of their power base. If Power = Resources × Importance × Scarcity, it can be seen how *Consultant B*'s interest group had come to corner so much power and influence.

Resources
Consultant B controlled resources in terms of money and academic influence. Charge Nurse F controlled resources in terms of staffing and trade union power, being a local shop steward in the union to which most of the nurses belonged.

Scarcity
Consultant B was the only doctor with experience of the specialist care of patients undergoing certain specialist interventions, a growing part of the unit's work. *Charge Nurse F* was the only senior nurse who had maintained an interest in new methods and new technology. He was thus the only nurse of this grade able to help when less experienced staff ran into difficulty. *Staff Nurse B* was the only member to have achieved a prestigious professional award in recent years.

As the factors mentioned with respect to resources and scarcity were obviously central to the survival of the unit, the source of power clearly lay with *Consultant B*'s group. It is said that the use of organisation theory is to provide a cognitive map of the subject under study. In this map all roads lead to *Consultant B*.

Effects of the change in the dominant coalition on staff

Changes in relationships

The ascendancy of *Consultant B* and her team caused marked differences in the way that the two consultants treated patients. This was particularly true in the case of children attending the specialist out-patient unit.

The care of children with chronic multi system diseases is rarely simple; a range of approaches is usually required, with the detailed management being tailored to the needs of each child and family. Senior nurses are often consulted about the balance between different types of care that is appropriate for a particular individual. As the change in the balance of power became more obvious, however, the views of the nurses on the unit were increasingly ignored, particularly by *Consultant A*. He altered management plans at short notice, exacerbating the tensions between those nursing and support staff loyal to him and those in the dominant coalition led by *Consultant B*.

Much of the responsibility for maintaining working relationships was borne by *Charge Nurse F*. As the trade union shop steward for nursing and support staff, he had to work closely with staff in the Specialist Out-patient Unit and on the ward. Uneasy but workable compromises were reached as a result of his personal efforts and attempts to maintain and improve professional standards. It became necessary, however, for him to maintain his role as crisis deflector for an extended period as power relationships within the unit took approximately three years to reach a new equilibrium. This prolonged period as the recipient of his colleagues' grievances as their main counsellor adversely affected his own commitment and eventually he resigned.

Staff turnover

As *Charge Nurse F* relinquished his role, *Staff Nurse B*, a rising star and powerful figure in *Consultant B*'s group, replaced him. A popular figure in the dominant coalition, he was promoted in preference to a member of *Consultant A*'s group who had greater experience in this field. The period of unrest resulted in an increased turnover of staff. Traditionally, turnover in the unit had been low, and at a fairly constant rate. The reason for leaving had predominantly been the 'pull' factors of professional advancement. Now, 'push' factors had come into play and staff left to escape the tension and conflict that the upheavals of the consultants' power struggle had created.

That such manifest changes in the power relationship within a unit were allowed to go unnoticed by the hospital management, particularly in view of the effects on staff, indicated the weakness of the systems used for monitoring the health of the organisation as a whole.

Longer-term effects on staff

The situation had taken several years to reach a new equilibrium. Some difficulties caused by the changes in the power relationship between the two consultants were due to *Consultant A*'s difficulty in redefining his role, in particular his area of influence. His enthusiasm for intensive care, for example, could have been used to develop and exploit his expert status. As his power base waned, he initially developed an interest in yet another area of paediatrics. Had this been pursued, his sessional commitment to the specialist out-patient unit could have been reduced. He could then have consolidated his in-patient power and increased his influence elsewhere. His enthusiasm for this other area was, however, short-lived, and he returned to his previous timetable and pattern of work.

However, an equilibrium had now been reached. *Consultant B* remained the dominant force but the loss of talented senior staff because of the unrest had increased her commitment to compromise and collaborative working. Similarly, *Consultant A* now had a more measured approach to his work, being less likely to amend long-term management plans in order to carry out new treatments about which he was enthusiastic. The potentially beneficial aspects of the complementary way in which *Consultants A* and *B* worked were recognised clearly by all parties when a third consultant, a locum, was appointed on a time-limited basis as a result of a regional initiative. This appointment highlighted the need for all groups of staff to work together to ensure the success of the unit and secure its future as part of the new Trust Hospital.

Effects of the change in the dominant coalition on patients

Whilst it may not be desirable, it is common for children with chronic diseases to become dependent on members of the specialist team who care for them. The patients attending this unit were no different. The patients and their families, therefore, like the staff, fell into three groups: those who were loyal to *Consultant A*, those who were loyal to *Consultant B* and those who had no firm allegiance to either. Patients loyal to *Consultant A* tended to be older, and either had milder disease or had undergone treatment in the intensive care unit for an acute illness. The style of practice favoured by the two camps also varied; *Consultant A*'s patients preferred a more traditional, hierarchical relationship. *Consultant B*'s approach was more like a partnership with the patient and the family. As well as younger children with more severe symptoms, she also attracted most of the female adolescent patients.

The chronic nature of patients' conditions meant that over the years patients were cared for by the consultant with whom they had developed the closest and most constructive relationship, despite the first choice of their general practitioners when making the original request for help with their management. As a result, whilst new patients and their families were subjected to several disruptive and inconvenient changes in both the nature and the style of their treatment, established patients were protected from the worst of the friction between the consultants and the nursing and support staff.

Over a period of six to nine months, however, the change in the dominant coalition began to have an effect on the way that the unit was run and clinical decisions made. Traditionally, the unit had been managed as *Consultant A* had developed it. This entailed an individualistic approach to patients. The treatments he prescribed, whilst their appropriateness could not be challenged on purely medical grounds, varied widely between patients. This meant that lessons learned from treating one patient could not be easily applied by staff to a similar situation involving another patient. It could not be assumed that *Consultant A* would react in the same way to the same clinical situation two days running. This inconsistency made it difficult for the nursing staff on the specialist unit to use their skills to their full potential; it is difficult to prepare patients for a clinical procedure or treatment if it is impossible, even for an experienced charge nurse or sister, to predict what it will be.

The ascendancy of the dominant coalition led by *Consultant B* led gradually to a more standardised approach to care being introduced. Guidelines, to assist nursing and junior medical staff in prioritising and choosing treatment options and preparing patients appropriately, were developed. Ways of standardising the quality of care received by different types of patient were also introduced.

In the short term, during the period of greatest unrest, it is likely that the care of patients, particularly patients new to the specialist out-patient unit, was less than perfect. The new equilibrium has, however, led to improvements in all aspects of care, both clinical and organisational.

Conclusions

The change in power relationships in the Unit described in this Case Study was not the consequence of planning or the direct intervention of the management level above the Unit. On the contrary, it took place informally and over a relatively long period. Such informal, partly hidden, processes are indicative of how much management change is achieved. They can lead ultimately to positive consequences for an organisation, as happened in the Paediatric Unit, but there is no guarantee that they will and, as we have seen, they can also bring with them hidden costs as in the damage inflicted on staff morale, leading to increased turnover, and in the adverse impact on patient care. The new and apparently beneficial equilibrium established in the Unit by the end of the Case Study came about partly because of the salutary effect of the loss of good staff of both consultants, as well as from the appointment of an additional (part-time) consultant which made *Consultants A* and *B* think long and hard about their relationship and the future of the Unit.

A responsible organisation, it might be thought, should not have to leave the outcomes of such conflicts to chance, nor simply accept their costs as inevitable. Arguably, it would be better for everyone involved in organisations such as the Unit if the staff become more organisationally self-conscious. In particular, doctor-managers need to give more time to gaining an understanding of the organisations they are working in and the dynamic of the interpersonal relationships that hold them together. In this way they may become more critically aware of what is happening much earlier in episodes such as that described in this Case Study, and be better-placed to act speedily and constructively in resolving the issues at stake.

Change

Introduction

Change is an unavoidable part of modern organisational life as even the first three studies dealing with equilibrium demonstrate. The cases presented in this final section, however, all focus on organisations which made deliberate attempts to introduce changes to improve their methods of operation. The first (Case Study 7) illustrates the ability of an entrenched group of professional workers to resist innovations. The next study (Case Study 8) shows how the members of an organisation can learn from the experience of a partial failure to introduce change. The last two studies (Case Studies 9 and 10) describe the conditions in which successful change was achieved but also illustrate how difficult it is to anticipate unintended consequences of the best laid plans.

Case Study 7: Resistance to change in an Obstetrics Unit

A Senior House Officer

Editors' introduction
The obstetrics unit which is the focus of this study was moderately large and busy, in that there were about 2,000 deliveries per year. It was also recognised for training purposes. The setting is an interesting one in that it is atypical of the conventional nurse–doctor model. That is to say, the relationship of the midwives to the junior doctors (SHOs) involved does not follow the Victorian ethos of nursing from the Nightingale era in which nurses assist doctors and remain largely subservient to medical staff (Garmarnikow, 1978; Porter, 1991). This type of atypical relationship between doctors and nurses has also been described in casualty units. Three factors were identified in casualty units which appeared to

contribute to the increased power of nurses. Firstly, the volume of cases to be treated was very large; too many to be seen initially by medical staff. Secondly, the turnover of medical staff was high relative to that of nursing staff and, for this reason, an inexperienced doctor sought help and advice from skilled and experienced nurses. Thirdly, the nursing staff were more likely to be from the local area and sensitive to the social cues from the patients (Hughes, 1988). In the study described here, the first two factors, and possibly the third, are present in the obstetrics unit as in casualty departments. The Case Study reveals that the skills of the midwives in diagnosis and treatment in most of the routine situations gives them authority in relationship to the SHOs. However, the relationship between the consultants and the registrar on the one hand and the midwives on the other is of a different nature, in which the doctors retain power, based on their expertise, particularly in difficult obstetric situations.

Another theme concerns that of change management and perhaps how it should not be carried out. A good idea for change, that of introducing a midwife from outside the unit in order to promote in staff a greater understanding of mothers' needs and greater patient choice in the way confinements and deliveries were handled, is resisted. The analysis reveals that no prior thought had been given to the likely countervailing forces of support or resistance in the unit and the values underlying the latter. The change agent (the new midwife), with little power is injected into the situation in isolation and the momentum for change is lost.

Organisational perspectives: the emphasis on the difference which can emerge between hierarchies of power and authority (Introduction, page 23) provides the main explanatory thrust of this study. It shows how such disparities can lead to particular problems where those with power (here, the midwives on the labour ward) successfully evade responsibilities that would logically be attached to that power, while those without effective power (the SHOs) retain them. The study also provides insight into how power at lower levels of an organisation can emerge and become consolidated from a concentration of professional expertise at those levels and the lack of proactive management above them.

The Case Study

This Case Study looks at the experience of five newcomers to an obstetrics unit. It will examine the needs and objectives of these five actors, their interaction with the obstetric unit and, by considering the outcomes of these interactions, it will outline how medical training, the practice of midwifery and staff interaction within the unit could be improved.

Setting the scene

Before such analysis can take place it is necessary to describe the stage on which the action is to take place. The obstetrics unit under consideration is part of an average sized District General Hospital and has an organisational structure composed of two professional bureaucracies, one medical and one nursing. These are summarised in Diagram 2.21, below.

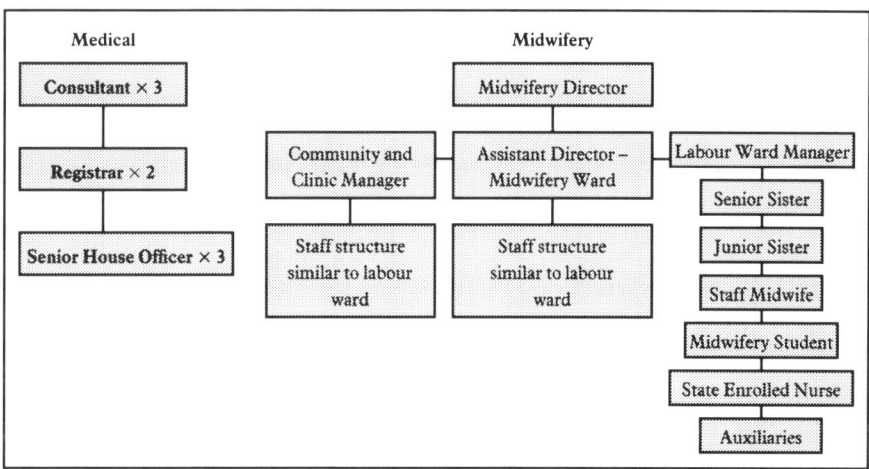

Diagram 2.21 Formal organisation of the Obstetrics Unit

In any bureaucracy power and influence tend to increase as you move up the hierarchy. In the obstetrics unit this was the case on the medical side. However, on the midwifery side most of the power was concentrated partway up the hierarchy in the hands of the labour ward manager and sisters. The labour ward was dominant over the rest of the unit (wards and clinics), with everything usually revolving around its functions. To consider the medical and nursing 'units' as separate entities is somewhat artificial as they are intimately intermingled in the day-to-day running of the unit. The relative distribution of power and influence between the doctors and midwives will be considered later.

The primary task of the unit could be regarded as effective care (as defined by the doctors and midwives) of pregnant women throughout their pregnancy. Both the medical and midwifery 'sides' also had a commitment to teach and train staff. Beyond this, the midwives were very committed to establishing the importance of the role of the midwife as a practitioner.

The actors

Four of the newcomers to the unit were doctors, three Senior House Officers and one Registrar. Their individual characteristics, needs and expectations will now be explored.

The Registrar was a career obstetrician and was technically and theoretically competent. He also had good interpersonal skills which he frequently used to his advantage. It could be said that he had perfected the hospital doctor career game – how to be seen at all the right times, how to take all the credit on offer but none of the blame and, most importantly, how to flatter the consultants. As he was a career obstetrician he was motivated by the job itself. His main objectives from the attachment were to gain good practical experience and to impress the consultants and thereby obtain a good reference.

Senior House Officer 1 This doctor was thinking about a career in obstetrics and already had accumulated quite a lot of obstetric experience, in fact, he could already perform most of the procedures expected of an SHO. He tended to be frank, open and honest and had a questioning/confrontational nature. His main objectives were to receive further training and experience in obstetrics. If the attachment was enjoyable it was to be used as a stepping stone to a future career in obstetrics.

Senior House Officer 2 was a general practice trainee with wide previous medical experience. Some thought him to be a little arrogant at work. He usually worked on the doctor–nurse model (ie doctors doctor and nurses nurse) and like *SHO1* he also tended to be questioning and confrontational. His objectives were to obtain the necessary experience and training which would allow him to be confident when dealing with obstetric conditions in general practice and to be 'accredited' by the Royal College of General Practitioners as having successfully completed six months training in obstetrics.

Senior House Officer 3 was also a general practice trainee. He was quiet, likeable and not one to make his grievances widely known. He was more accepting and compliant than the other SHOs. His objective was primarily to see the six months through with the minimum amount of trouble, any training and experience being an added bonus.

The Midwife Our final actor is in fact an actress, a midwife. She trained in an area outside the district and had gained a wide experience of midwifery in many different units. She was accustomed to the practice of progressive midwifery and to having a high degree of responsibility in the care of her women. She was open and honest and gave respect when it was due and not because of someone's position. Her objectives were to practice midwifery, earn money and to be happy in her work. She was told at the start of her job that she was expected to expose the midwives working in the unit to different ideas and methods of practice.

The outcome of the interaction between the actors and the obstetric unit

The interrelationship of the doctors and midwives in the unit and its outcome will be considered in two sections, the training and educational needs of the four doctors and the needs of the unit.

Training and educational needs

These were shared by all the doctors. Although being recognised by the Joint Committee for Higher Medical Training for both Registrar and GP training, the unit gave a very low priority to such education and training. There was no training policy or programme within the unit, and no one consultant was given the responsibility for dealing with training issues. The consultants possibly thought that the Registrars were carrying out more training than they actually were. In common with many junior medical jobs, the need to perform the routine work far outweighed any training or educational needs. The Registrar was least affected by this as he already had acquired the basic knowledge needed in his post. What he now required was more practical experience and in the unit he was receiving a plentiful supply. Some training was given to the SHOs in the first few weeks of the attachment, mostly by the Registrars, not the Consultants. This training was as much for the benefit of the Registrars themselves as for the SHOs, as once the SHOs knew enough to perform the routine procedures the training stopped.

The lack of training soon began to lead to dissatisfaction amongst the SHOs and their morale suffered as a consequence. Often the lack of training in a medical job can be offset by the satisfaction and pleasure that doing a good job (and being acknowledged for doing so) can bring. In situations where there is very little training, a good working environment becomes particularly crucial to maintaining staff morale.

The needs of the unit

In considering the working of the unit, it is important to realise that as well as the actors having needs, the organisation – or more accurately, those responsible for managing it – needs to socialise (or coerce) new members to performing tasks in the accepted manner, and to acknowledge the rules and regulations of the organisation. The first part of this section will consider the interaction between the unit and the new doctors and the second part the interaction between the unit and the midwife.

The doctors. Communication and interaction between the doctors was poor. There was very little direct interaction between the Consultants and the SHOs and it was often left to the Registrars to make such links between them as they could. Communication was also poor between the Consultants themselves. As a result of all this the SHOs were denied the sense of belonging to a team and had very little positive feedback on their performance. Their morale deteriorated further.

Of particular significance in terms of the training needs of the SHOs was the nature of their interaction with the midwives and the power struggle that developed between the two groups. The midwives were very keen on being seen as independent practitioners and in addition to this the labour ward staff as a whole appeared to want to defend their territory against medical 'intruders'. The doctors, on the other hand, were used to having the upper hand in the power struggle with nurses and tended to want to take over the responsibility for decision making. However, this expectation was somewhat modified in the case of obstetrics by comparison with the situation found in general wards in that the midwives have specialised skills and knowledge, and most doctors would be willing to allow them some autonomy provided that they also accept responsibility for their decisions.

The overall distribution of power and responsibility between doctors and nurses which developed in practice in the unit are shown in Diagram 2.22 below.

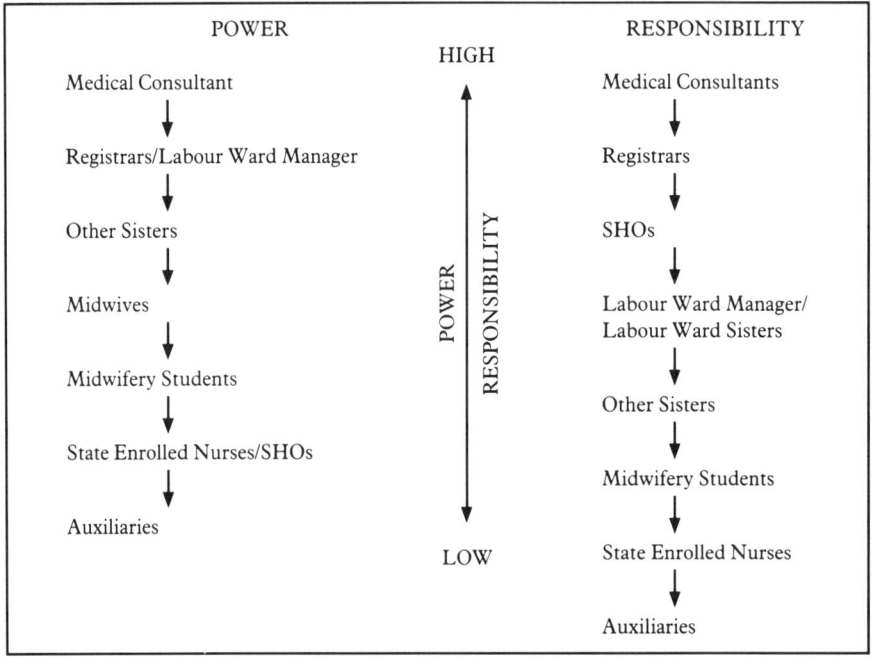

Diagram 2.22 Power and responsibility in the Labour Ward

It can be seen that the midwives were prepared to accept more power than responsibility thereby reducing the legitimacy of their claim to be independent practitioners. In contrast to the midwives, the junior doctors had relatively more responsibility than power which often caused them much frustration as they felt they were responsible for making decisions, but did not have the necessary power to institute them. What was happening, in effect, was that the midwives were only contacting the SHOs over cases because they 'had' to according to the formal procedures of the unit. When they disagreed with their opinions, however, they either ignored them completely or contacted the Registrar for his views. It might be argued that this was 'wise' practice as midwives should have more experience of obstetrics than junior doctors but the effect on the SHOs was to make them feel frozen out. It seemed that they existed merely to do the routine work and act as a communication channel between the midwives and the Registrars, rather than being involved in the care of pregnant women. This dissonance between power and responsibility, added to the other factors (lack of training, feedback and teamwork), made the SHOs feel exploited and frustrated.

The hierarchy of power which achieved this result had been arrived at by conflict and negotiation, with all the trump cards being held by the midwives. The power struggle had reached its peak on the labour ward but was maintained throughout the unit. *SHOs 1* and *2* had attempted to maintain some power at first, but were soon to accept their position when the midwives began to make their lives intolerable. *SHO 3* had been prepared to accept this position from the outset and as a result had a much easier ride.

The Consultants and Registrars were not involved in the battle as their position as the experts was recognised and legitimised by the midwives and their lack of regular contact with the SHOs meant they had little idea of the nature of their working relationships with the midwives. Ward rounds often took place without the SHOs being present, and work in consultant clinics was infrequent. The SHOs were attached to wards and not Consultants which also reduced contact. The Consultants were probably unaware of the training grievances of the SHOs as the working environment did not encourage open discussions of that nature. The routine work commitments of the SHOs was high which further restricted the possibility of training sessions.

In summary all the SHOs felt exploited and that they got the credit for very little whilst they appeared to be blamed for everything. All agreed that this was the worst medical appointment they had ever experienced. This conclusion was not a unique one to this group as the SHOs before and after this attachment all felt the same. None of the SHOs felt that his training/educational needs had been fulfilled. The Registrar, in contrast, met all his objectives and, as he was not involved in the power struggle, enjoyed the attachment.

The midwife. Most of the midwives working on the unit had also trained there and had little experience of practice elsewhere. This made the unit very insular, resistant to change and suspicious of 'outsiders'. To succeed in the unit a midwife had to be liked by the dominant midwives (labour ward staff) and follow the accepted rules. Midwives were either socialised into accepting the rules and dominant values or left the unit. In this way the unit 'selected' those midwives that would maintain the *status quo*. The rules and regulations of the unit (originating mainly from the labour ward) were made clear to the new midwife from day one – 'We do things this way here, not like that!'. Any procedures and practices that were unusual or contrary to the accepted practice were immediately identified and the necessary sanctions taken.

It had been the idea of the Director of Midwifery Services to introduce new blood into the unit so that the practice of midwifery could be invigorated. The Director of Midwifery was on paper the most powerful midwife on the unit, but in reality the labour ward manager and staff were dominant. The new midwife, therefore, without the backing of a powerful ward level manager, stood very little chance of introducing new practice, as soon became clear. She was often isolated by the senior staff and given women to look after who were post-natal rather than in labour. She came to feel that her practice was being interfered with, and that the other experienced midwives were constantly watching over her and did not trust her. She was often told that she was doing things which were not regarded as common practice on the unit, but these 'rules' were never written down and appeared to be known only to the senior staff. Her opinions on practice, which she expressed at midwifery meetings, were typically disregarded, usually without discussion. Many of the younger midwives were interested in these opinions and discussed them at length afterwards, but none of them was confident enough to do so during the meetings in front of the senior staff. In all these ways she was prevented from ever feeling part of the team, but instead was treated as a dangerous radical who had to be made to toe the line. This was in direct opposition to the original aims of the Director of Midwifery who had employed her in the hope that she would bring outside experience into the unit and move the practice of midwifery there forward.

As the midwife was used to practising progressive midwifery and to accepting responsibility for her decisions, she found it hard to cope with the constant haranguing she received for what she considered was routine good practice. She felt that she could not practice her profession under these restrictions and left the unit for another position.

This culture of resistance to change was not reserved solely for new members of staff but was also extended to the pregnant mothers. If they did not wish to follow the 'normal' method of delivery they were treated with disdain and made to feel uncomfortable. This was perhaps the biggest indictment of the whole unit.

Conclusions and suggestions for improvement.

We have seen that out of the five actors only one could be said to have had a successful outcome, the Registrar. The SHOs were demoralised by the end of the attachment and felt that they had achieved very little. The lack of a training/educational component and lack of team spirit were the main failings on the medical side. It is difficult to see how the situation could change without the primary task of the unit incorporating a training element. The routine service work will still predominate since there is no real incentive for change thanks to the plentiful supply of doctors looking for obstetric attachments. However, if the regulatory bodies who are responsible for continuing medical education were to become more active and critical of training locations and took into account the views of previous doctors some impetus for change could develop. Improved inter-Consultant and Consultant–SHO communication would also help the SHOs to feel more involved in the work of the unit. It would also allow a more receptive culture to develop in which grievances could be freely aired, thereby allowing the Consultants to appreciate fully the importance of good quality training and good staff morale.

Possible solutions would be to establish a training programme for SHOs with one of the Consultants being made responsible for its implementation. A change to a system whereby each SHO is attached to a Consultant would also improve team work and allow more opportunities for training. The underlying problem of the very high level of routine work in this post would make it difficult to implement any substantial training programme without any further increase in SHO numbers. Improved liaison between the Consultants and the midwives would help foster better doctor–midwife relationships which would lessen the power struggle as both groups began to understand one another. Such a change would need to be initiated by the Consultants and senior midwives if it is to succeed. All policies and accepted practice guidelines should be recorded and subject to constant review.

The experience of the new midwife is perhaps the most worrying. It demonstrates how rigid and inflexible the current unit is. In order to improve the situation within the midwifery unit it would appear that the dominance of the labour ward has to be broken. This could be achieved by increasing the rotation of midwives through the labour ward from the other parts of the unit and by appointing (and retaining) more staff from outside the area. A consensus culture between midwife and midwife, and between midwife and doctor, would take some time to develop fully, but would be well worth working towards as the improved staff morale would be welcome news for those working within the unit as well as for the patients. Eventually the pregnant mothers themselves might become involved in this consensus culture and be allowed to play a full and rewarding part in their own pregnancies.

Case Study 8: Learning from failure: The introduction of a practice nurse

A General Practitioner

Editors' introduction

This study of a general practice provides a cogent example of how an intended improvement in organisation can have unintended, dysfunctional consequences. It also illustrates how the same organisation can learn from its mistakes and even turn them to its advantage. The practice partners show considerable prescience in recognising that change in their practice will be required if they are to achieve not only the best for their patients, but also respond to the provision of services being recommended by relevant professional organisations. Responding, for example, to the suggestions and drive for preventive care in practice populations in publications of the Royal College of General Practitioners, in addition to reacting to the direct demands of patients. This foresight has since been confirmed by the subsequent new contract for General Practice in which many procedures such as screening for disease, surveillance of the elderly and other preventive programmes are linked to payment of GPs (Department of Health and the Welsh Office, 1989).

The practice described had achieved a comfortable equilibrium based on good personal relationships between the various professional (GP, district nurse and health visitor) and support staff groups. The instigation for change, namely the introduction of a practice nurse to take responsibility for a screening service and follow-up clinics for chronic diseases, came from the GP partners (the dominant coalition) but was implemented within the consultative style of management prevailing in the practice. The Case Study shows nicely how the various professional and other groups within the practice weighed up the costs and benefits to their own group and their responses. Resistance to the change arose largely after implementation rather than in response to the idea itself, and the perceived objectives of the change. This resistance manifested itself mainly in the form of the use of negative power by the district nurse and health visitor groups. In reaction to the problems raised by the practice nurse's approach to screening, the GP partners moved towards a more participative mode of management within the practice. Thus, the planned change in practice procedures has in itself produced a change or adaptation in the management style of the GP partners. This begs the question of whether any organisation contemplating a change, particularly in size or complexity of subsystems should in advance address the question of whether its current mode of management is equal to the task.

Organisational perspectives: this Case Study uses an open systems model (Introduction, pages 25–6) to provide the overall framework of analysis. This approach effectively identifies the tasks which the general practitioners must achieve to enable their practice to survive and flourish. It is also valuable in defining the nature of the links between the different groups (or subsystems) within the organisation and in evaluating the implications of the arrival of the practice nurse for these interrelationships. In explaining the different perspectives of the members of the various subsystems, an action approach is used (Introduction, pages 28–9) to good effect to expose the contrasting views and interests of their members. The evolving management style of the general practitioners, moving from a consultative to a more participative approach, is explored in terms of concepts developed in the neo-human relations literature (Introduction, pages 26–8).

The Case Study

A few years ago a three man, health centre-based, general practice decided, because of pressure from outside the organisation, to add to its primary goal – satisfying enough patients to maintain the practice list size to ensure viability – the mission task of improving the overall health of the practice population. This was to be achieved by providing an increased number of screening procedures for the patients in order to identify the unmet need for services, the provision of those services thus identified, and the more efficient use of those services already provided by the practice. The existing structure of the organisation was thought to be unable to cope with the inevitable increase in workload as a result of such change. Possible solutions to cope with the proposed change were considered. It was felt that the most acceptable solution was to employ a practice nurse.

The structure of the Practice: An open systems model

The organisation could have been considered to operate in the fashion of an open system with characteristics in common with a biological organism that is existing by exchanging materials, goods or services with the environment. The imports to the system were those members of the practice population either with a problem or were those being screened for a problem. The transformation process consisted of all those activities within the organisation concerned with patient care. The desired exports were those patients satisfied as a result of their contact with the organisation. Those satisfied patients provided the necessary feedback into the system to ensure its viability both by reattending with the same or a different problem themselves or, more importantly, by encouraging others to sign on to the practice list because of their own satisfaction with the service provided by the organisation. This was effected by local word of mouth (see Diagram 2.23). At this stage the organisation's primary task was to survive and to maximise profit to ensure a reasonable income for the partners.

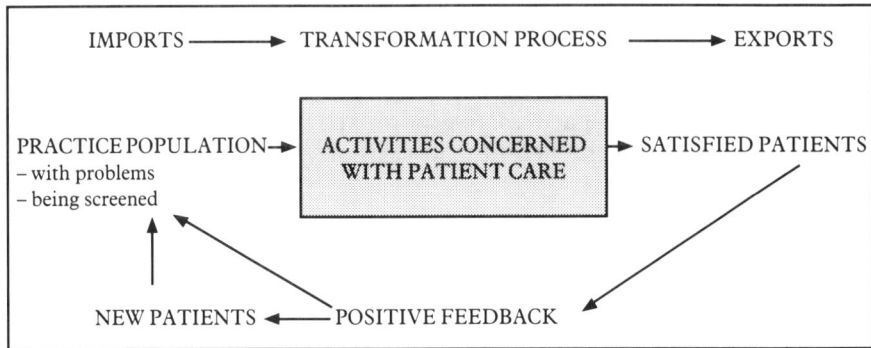

Diagram 2.23   The organisation as a system

Systems of activity and boundaries

The operating activities, or those activities directly concerned with the import, transformation and export process of the practice, would have been all those activities directed towards attracting patients, providing services for them and effecting patient satisfaction with those services in order to encourage the feedback essential to maintain patient flow and hence the survival of the organisation.

The maintenance activities, or those activities which ensure the replenishment of the resources necessary to enable the operating activities of the practice to continue, would have been those concerned with maintaining staff numbers at a level sufficient to deliver effective services, maintenance of the fabric of the health centre and the provision of sufficient equipment to enable service provision.

Since the practice operated from a health centre the responsibility for the operating and maintenance activities was shared by the partners and the health authority in some instances, and it was not always clear where the responsibility lay, or should continue to lie in certain instances. For example, the responsibility for the maintenance of the fabric of the building lay with the health authority, the partners paying appropriate rent. This responsibility remained quite clear.

However, the district nursing service, provided by the health authority, was required to provide a minimum service to the patients of the practice list as instructed by the partners. Any duties over and above this minimum were negotiated as favours which rapidly became accepted as routine, thereby blurring the boundaries between the roles of the district nurse and the doctor. With the move towards the extended role of the district nurse it became unclear as to who was responsible for the continuing provision of these previously negotiated services. This was brought to light when the district nurses were asked by the partners to administer influenza vaccine to some elderly persons at home because of their difficulty in attending the surgery. The nurses were advised by their manager that this request was not acceptable since the risk of adverse reaction to the vaccine required a doctor to be present at its administration. However, the nurses had for many years given other injections which carried a similar risk of reaction, both in the surgery and at patient's homes, without a doctor being present or readily available. A similar situation existed between the health visitors and the doctors.

The regulatory activities relating the activities within the organisation to each other, and the activities within the practice to the external environment, were of a largely informal nature in that there were very few clearly defined boundaries and even defined boundaries were often breached as discussed above. However, further discussion will confirm that these boundaries were already becoming more clearly defined prior to the appointment of the practice nurse.

The subsystems

The organisation was composed of several subsystems, each contributing a particular expertise in an autonomous fashion. The general practice partnership subsystem, acting as the dominant coalition, regulated the activities, in most instances, between the boundaries of the subsystems and between the organisation and the external environment. The practice partnership held the formal authority to manage and direct the organisation as a whole by dint of the expert power of each of the partners. The subsystems of the organisation which are relevant to consider in this analysis are the:

General Practice partnership, reception and secretarial staff, district nursing service and the health visiting service.

The General Practice partnership

The general practice partnership had existed for four years. The two, male, senior, full-time partners had worked together for twelve years prior to the arrival of the replacement, female, junior, part-time partner. Each of the partners worked independently of one another operating with a common practice list. However, the formation of a consensus of approach was beginning. The female partner had had some reservations about the variety of treatments and treatment combinations prescribed by the practice partners for some conditions. Initially informal discussions over coffee resulted in some rationalisation of prescribing across the partnership. The repeat prescription system became less complex as a result of this, kindling an interest in discussing further prescribing rationalisation. A local hospital physician was approached to facilitate further discussion in this area and monthly meetings between the partners and the physician were about to begin.

With the murmurings of change both in general and hospital practice towards more choice for the consumer, the partnership began in 1988 to look to instigate those services which would eventually be required of them, and therefore of the organisation, by pressure from the external environment. With outside commitments the partnership felt unable to absorb the inevitable increase in workload which would result from the provision of these services and since both the district nursing and health visiting services were either unwilling, or too overworked to take on the extra services, the decision to employ a practice nurse was made. This was seen as the most cost-effective way for the partnership to provide the additional services.

The reception and secretarial staff

This subsystem consisted of two receptionists who had worked together for seven years and a secretary who had been working with them for three years. The roles of these three members were interchangeable with one of the receptionists taking the lead responsibility for financial matters. The only member with any appropriate training was the secretary. However, these members of staff were graded as equal from a payscale viewpoint and were employed by the practice partnership. This group of staff was essential to the smooth operation of the organisation, acting as a co-ordinating body, liaising between the patients, district nurses, health visitors and doctors. Its members were often caught in the middle of disagreements and their importance was underestimated, particularly by the partners. Their reward was small and their loyalty impressive. The reason for this loyalty may well have lain in the fact that this task group was also a strong 'sentient' group, sharing values and feelings.

The reception and secretarial staff were very receptive to the ideal of the new mission task of improving the overall health of the practice population, not least because they were all patients of the practice. They saw a practice nurse as a doctor substitute and felt, therefore, that more patients could be seen thereby reducing the number of confrontations they might have with patients because of a lack of appointments with the doctors. They saw the inevitable increase in their own workload as a result of such an appointment as being outweighed by the advantages.

The District Nursing Service

The district nursing service subsystem consisted of a district nursing sister, a state enrolled nurse and a bath attendant. Although they were all health authority employees their duties were specific to the practice partnership. The partnership had no control over the appointment of these individuals but delegated appropriate work to them or negotiated favours as necessary.

As was the case in other nursing services the district nursing service was itself undergoing change at the time. More administrative duties were becoming the order of the day and there was a tightening in the level of responsibility allowable for any given nurse. For example, tasks which had been undertaken unsupervised in the past were no longer allowed. The district nurses were therefore becoming less willing to accept delegation, whilst at the same time wanting to protect the importance of their role. Discussion with the district nurses on the delegation of tasks implied in the additional services which would result from the adoption of the new mission task of the organisation, was met with resistance.

The Health Visiting Service

Two health visitors and a health visitor assistant made up the members of this subsystem. They were all health authority employees and were shared between the partnership and a single handed general practitioner who was also based at the health centre. The partnership had no involvement in the appointment of these staff and were very much reliant on their voluntary cooperation. As a group they were rather more autonomous than the district nurses and had their own remit of work from the health authority.

Cooperation had always been very good between the doctors and the health visitors but the changes described in the relationship between the district nurses and the doctors seemed to be infectious as far as this group were concerned. The health visitors' attitude, despite the fact that part of their remit is concerned with health promotion, was

'by all means increase screening procedures but we have too much work to do as it is to be part of them.'

The relationship between the subsystems of the organisation

Within the individual subsystems the relationships between the members were good, with task and sentient groups coinciding. Between the subsystems, despite changes being enforced from the external environment, the relationships were generally good, but there were perhaps signs that these relationships might not be as good in the future. However, since the primary goal and mission task were common to, and accepted by, all the subsystems and because sentient groups overlapped the subsystem boundaries there were hopes that good relationships would continue.

A diagrammatic representation of the avenues of patient progress through the organisation emphasises the interrelationship of the subsystems (see Diagram 2.24). Up until the beginning of the change within the organisation the boundaries between the areas of patient care of each subsystem were not always clear. A great deal of overlap of care occurred as a result of the good interpersonal relationships between the actors of each of the subsystems. As a result of the lack of clearly defined roles,

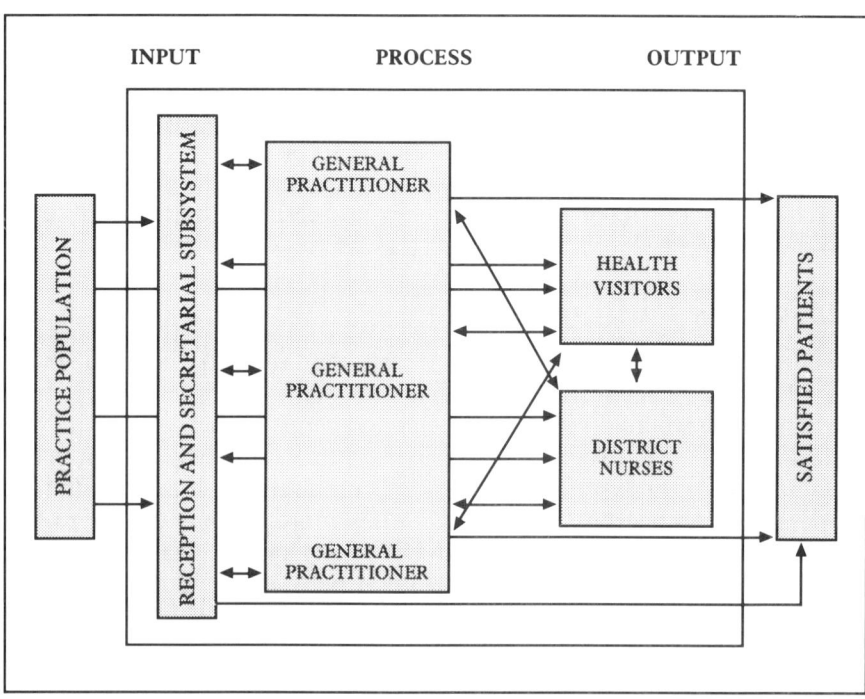

Diagram 2.24 Patient progress through the system and the interrelationship of the subsystems

occasional role stress occurred, which could be either beneficial or harmful to the organisation depending on the particular situation, and which was resolved by negotiation between the parties concerned. The relative stability of the organisation had therefore developed without an explicit need for written documents defining variables such as the partnership agreement, individual job descriptions, conditions of employment or procedure policies.

Although all actions concerned with the care of a patient registered with the practice partnership were the ultimate responsibility of the individual general practitioner, members of each of the subsystems were encouraged to take responsibility, within their own capability, and to consult with their own superior or one of the general practitioners for advice as appropriate. Most of the members of each of the subsystems had their own professional authority and/or motivation towards self actualisation. There was, however, a hierarchy within each of the subsystems relating to each individual's power. This resulted as a consequence of that individual's relative expert power within their own subsystem and their length of service. The presence of these hierarchies had a tendency to complicate the management strategies of the dominant coalition. A consultative approach to decision making (as defined by Likert's System 3 model of management) would most closely describe how the dominant coalition operated from a management point of view, although the results of consultation seemed, all too often, to be the views of the dominant coalition.

The introduction of the Practice Nurse

The person appointed as the part-time practice nurse, from a shortlist of five, was an experienced State Registered Nurse who had worked in responsible positions in hospitals abroad and was used to working on her own initiative. She had experience of screening populations for disease and of delivering health education. However, she had no general practice experience or recent experience of the health service in this country. Despite these gaps she was seen as having potential and projected herself in a manner thought to be appropriate to the character of the practice partnership.

In the practice she was expected to help in the setting up, and eventually taking over the responsibility for the running of, screening clinics and follow-up clinics for chronic diseases with a view to the delegation of other tasks, such as vaccinations, as deemed appropriate by the partnership at some stage in the future. These tasks were discussed at length prior to and following her appointment. She saw no difficulties with these expectations of her.

As was the fashion of the practice no formal agreements were drawn up in writing. This applied both to a job description and a contract of employment. A salary at the lower end of the recommended Whitley Payscale was negotiated and agreed.

Operational problems and their attempted solution

It had been envisaged by the practice partnership that the practice nurse would establish a separate subsystem which would take most of its input from the partners, at least initially. As time went by it was thought that those tasks which had been done as favours in the past by the district nurses and health visitors would find their way to the practice nurse. In reality all such patients were directed to the practice nurse by the members of the subsystems concerned as soon as she arrived. The practice nurse soon became overloaded and decided that she would only take referrals from the partners. As a result of this action both the district nurses and health visitors referred back to the partners those patients for whom they had been providing services as favours. The employment of the practice nurse thus resulted in the loss of goodwill between the partners and the district nurses and health visitors in relation to the tasks previously done as favours, and had increased the partners' workload as a consequence. This had been the very thing the partners had sought to avoid in employing a practice nurse.

It soon became obvious that the practice nurse's expectation of her role was not that expected of her by her new colleagues and, since her role had not been enshrined in a job description, ambiguity and confusion ensued. One of the partners was able to resolve some of the role ambiguity by prolonged discussion with the practice nurse, the district nurses and the health visitors. Unfortunately a degree of incompatibility remained in that the practice nurse's expectations of the standard of service achievable were not practicable within the constraints of the operation of the practice partnership. For example, her expectation was that any patient seen by her for whatever reason should have immediate access to a doctor for anything she was unable to deal with, whether the problem was apparently serious or trivial. This was a reflection of the practice nurse's lack of recent experience of health care in this country and in general practice in particular. She persisted with her views despite a very frank discussion involving all the doctors.

The stress which resulted as a consequence of the loss of goodwill between the partners and the district nurses and health visitors, the increased workload of the partners, and the role incompatibility of the practice nurse affected the relationship between all the subsystems and between the members of each of the subsystems in a detrimental fashion. Cooperation became a thing of the past. The organisation was in crisis.

The district nurses and health visitors refused to do anything more than was required of them as directed by their senior officers (who were based at the health authority headquarters). Other members of the organisation, nevertheless, tried to deal with the situation by remaining outwardly calm and polite. In contrast, the practice nurse exacerbated the situation by her behaviour. Her feelings of stress were expressed as irritation, excessive preoccupation with detail and stereotyped responses which all increased her sensitivity to the organisation's pressure on her to conform.

Eventually her low morale led to open expressions of dissatisfaction with the job and gradually communications between her and the organisation were confined to the bare minimum necessary for her to do her work. Her coping strategy changed as time went by. Initially it was one of withdrawal which quickly became that of rationalisation, since she saw the alternative of leaving the organisation as an admission of defeat. However, conflict within the organisation was now explicit, and since other actors were questioning their own roles much more critically as a result of the stress generated, the organisation's ability to achieve the new mission task was in jeopardy.

It seemed reasonable to the practice partners to attempt to reconcile the difficulties that had occurred in the organisation as a result of their introduction into the organisation of the practice nurse. After consultation with the practice nurse, who expressed a desire to remain within the organisation despite the difficulties to date, it was decided that a meeting should be called at which a representative from each subsystem should be present in order to solve the difficulties between the subsystems. Meetings of the members of each of the subsystems were encouraged to enable discussion of the organisation's problems, the formulation of possible solutions and the election of a representative. It was also hoped that these meetings would begin the process of defining the roles of individual members within each of the subsystems. The subsystem meetings took place as did the representatives' meeting.

It soon became clear that although the organisation had been able to operate in the past in a *laissez-faire* manner which had been highly dependent on good interpersonal relationships, the demands from the external environment and the increasing number of actors which were, and would in the future, be involved made it less likely that the organisation could continue to depend on this approach for its effective operation. A round of meetings were therefore begun at both subsystem and organisation level to decide where boundaries were to be drawn.

These meetings were ongoing when the author resigned to begin training in Public Health Medicine. It was already clear that role definitions were to be enshrined in job descriptions which would help to delineate the boundaries of the roles between the subsystems and between the members of the subsystems.

Conclusion

It could be argued that more careful selection of the successful candidate for the post of practice nurse would have averted the crisis which was faced by the organisation as a result of the appointment. However, it is my view that it was inevitable, given the changes facing general practice at that time, that such a crisis was likely to occur at some stage in the practice described, since the new philosophy of health care will be less accommodating of a *laissez-faire* style of organisation. The stress created as a result of the practice nurse's appointment brought to the surface and made explicit all sorts of currents of dissatisfaction within the organisation. Her appointment merely acted as the catalyst to enable those dissatisfactions to be resolved. This was achieved by a move from an organisation reliant on informal interpersonal relationships for its stability and effectiveness to one dependant upon rigidly controlled boundaries as defined by job descriptions. I suspect that gradually the rigidity of the consequences of these documents will soften towards the rather more flexible nature of the previous arrangements.

All the actors expressed their opinions openly and contributed to the process of change. The present situation has resulted, therefore, from a participative input from all members of the organisation – involving the practice in a move from Likert's System 3 model of consultative management to his System 4 model of participative management (Likert, 1967). This may not be the long-term model of management for this organisation but its adoption is, for the time being, allowing the mission goals to be achieved.

Case Study 9: Organisational decay, conflict and change in a Group Practice

A General Practitioner

Editors' introduction
This Case Study has the advantage of considering the development of a practice over a number of years, combining on the one hand the treatment and caring functions of the practice and, on the other, the practice as a business. In many ways, the development of the practice parallels the turmoil experienced, and adjustments required, over time by commercial companies as they search for high quality in their field of endeavour. Even companies rated as having responsive management and concern for customers, such as IBM (Peters and Waterman, 1982) cannot rely on

stability over long periods of time – witness the problems experienced by this company in 1992/93. The Case Study emphasises that the efforts to achieve the perceived need for change in this practice were principally concentrated on the structural aspects of the practice premises and the configuration and distribution of practice staff. In addition to the relative lack of attention to the staff values, the desired change was also compromised by apparently unforeseen events, in particular the ill health of some of the practice partners. The relationship between stressors, whether they are in the physical environment of the job, in the nature of the job itself or in organisational issues surrounding the job, are complex (Holmes & Rahe, 1967; Cooper & Marshall, 1976; Jee & Reason, 1988). Nevertheless, in this Case Study, the possibility cannot be dismissed that the change and destabilisation reported in this organisation was linked in a causal manner with ill health.

Organisational perspectives: this is a classic example of organisational change driven by an incomplete conception of the system involved. Planning of the financial and technical aspects of the reorganisation were meticulous, but the impact of the changes involved on the social structure of the practice seems not to have been considered. The author's careful analysis of the power structure of the practice before change, and his delineation of a situation where most of the control of the organisation had, by default, been acquired by the senior partner, makes the consequences of the change in terms of the social system of the practice readily understandable. The management of the change was delegated to two younger doctors and the other doctors continued to adopt a passive role. Yet, given the type of organisation concerned (professional – see Introduction, page 22) the close participation of the medical team, and the involvement of other practice staff (following neo-human relations analysis – Introduction, pages 26–8) would have been the logical strategy to follow. In this way it would have been at least possible that the likely impact of the proposed changes on staff could have been anticipated, and planned for, and the coherence of the management of the practice maintained throughout.

The Case Study

'Change is the watchword of Progression. When We tire of well-worn ways, we seek for new. This restless craving in the souls of men Spurs them to climb, and seek the mountain view.'

Ellen Wheeler Wilcox
The Year Outgrows the Spring, St.5.

Introduction

I entered general practice at Yatchester from a university academic department with the warning of my professor ringing in my years – 'You'll soon get tired of writing EC10s' (prescriptions). However, having spent the majority of my life in the area, I had been delighted to accept an invitation to join the practice. Although the last part of my time in the practice was often strife-ridden and uncertain, the many years I was there have given immense pleasure and understanding. Becoming part of a community and knowing its intricacies and innermost secrets is a privilege accorded few but is characteristic of life as a family doctor. General practice is a stage for all life's emotions, and the breadth of that experience has been formative and enlightening.

Social context
Yatchester is a small town at the centre of an area of mixed industrial and residential settlements, separated by tracts of open country. The 'practice area' includes eight geographically and socially distinct communities, most of which are within a radius of three miles of Yatchester. The population served by the practice is about 18,000 and the practice has a virtual monopoly of medical care in the area. This, combined with the stability of the population provides a secure business basis for its work.

The history of the Yatchester and Medley Medical Practice

Before the Second World War the communities of Yatchester and Medley were served by six family doctors with surgeries traditionally based in doctors' homes.

The history of the practice can be defined in four distinct periods:
(1) Evolution – pre-NHS to 1973
(2) Stability – 1973–1985
(3) Change – 1985–1988
(4) Instability – 1988 onwards.

Evolution
Encouraged by Government policy, an incremental amalgamation of practice units led to the formation of the present group practice in 1964. From 1960, Yatchester was served by purpose built premises in the High Street, which remained in use until 1987. Little Yatchester and Medley continued to have surgeries based in doctors' houses until the provision of a Local Authority Health Centre in Medley heralded their closure amidst public outcry at centralisation of services. It is interesting that, even in

1964, it was reported that there was conflict over the title of Senior Partner, the two longest serving doctors each claiming their right to the role. In the event, the case to prevail was that of the doctor who could claim that he had founded the High Street practice which had ended up as the home of the partnership!

A final consolidation of medical services in the area occurred in 1973 when another doctor joined the group, bringing with him the remnants of a further outlying practice.

Stability
The period from 1973 to 1985 saw relative stability in the practice with an expansion to six partners in 1975, and the replacement of two retiring senior partners in 1979, marking the end of the pre-NHS era.

Change
Between 1985 and 1988 the practice faced its greatest challenges since the introduction of the National Health Service in 1948. Practice accommodation had become outdated and a review of organisational structure was required in response to the increasing workload of a 'deprived area', the strengthening of the consumer role, and the concurrent creation of a Primary Health Care Team. The management of this change and the associated conflict form the basis of the following critical review of the organisation.

Instability
Finally, although there were undoubted benefits from the changes, the practice was destabilised, and dramatic changes in staff jeopardised the provision of effective health care services at a time when general practice was experiencing a crisis consequent to the demands of the new GP Contract and the introduction of the NHS changes and Community Care Act.

A critical review of the practice organisation

The practice entered the 1980s much as it had done the previous two decades – with little vision and no stimulus for development. Change was perceived as a threat to stability and proposals were likely to be vetoed at senior level. To understand the underlying pressures for change it is necessary to review the organisation at that time.

Buildings
The main surgery premises, built in the 1960s, had become grossly inadequate for the demands placed upon them. The available accommodation provided only 25% of the floor area recommended in the Statement

of Fees and Allowances (para 51, Schedule 1[5]), and its general fabric was poor. The provision of only two consulting rooms restricted surgery times and contributed to a chronic shortage of appointments. 'Doubling up' on use of rooms increased conflict on availability when the inevitable delays occurred. Nursing facilities were confined to the 'middle room' which, although designated a treatment room, had the operational characteristics of a corridor. The patients were faced with a cramped, uninviting waiting room with drab decor and a tattered collection of redundant magazines. Seating was provided on wooden chairs and leatherette benches in regimental rows facing the reception desks. The volume of patient contacts, the incessant telephone and queues of patients waiting for prescriptions or appointments created a turbulent and chaotic atmosphere.

The record system had long since exceeded its capacity and ragged 'Lloyd George' envelopes bulged from drawers and were stacked everywhere, creating an air of untidiness and disorganisation. The reception desk itself offered little privacy to patients and the multiple roles expected of the receptionist increased stress, so that a highly charged atmosphere developed and it is little wonder that the system generated a barrage of complaints.

The receptionists were able to retreat for coffee to the 'common room' but competed for space with the doctors in a room also serving as a cloakroom, meeting room and store room. As a 'no-smoking' policy had been rejected, the room was permanently smoke-laden and it is perhaps a reflection of the chaos prevailing in the 'front shop' that it was regarded as a cosy retreat!

The Practice Manager's Office, which was cramped and spartan, had a single desk which was shared with a part-time secretary. The central heating system had long since decayed and the building was heated inadequately with a collection of electric heaters with little regard to efficiency. In contrast, the Branch Surgery at Medley was situated at a Local Authority Health Centre with adequate, spacious facilities and an ambience reflecting its resources.

Personnel

The organisation was dominated by the doctors, with the senior partner at its apex. Ancillary staff were in direct line management to the practice manager, although her title was a euphemism for an administrative function with little autonomy. The reception staff were mainly part-time married ladies from the local community, the majority having been loyal to the practice for many years. The senior receptionist, a full-time employee, deputised for the practice manager in her absence and her long-standing experience made her an indispensible employee. The reception staff controlled access to the doctor and repeat prescriptions, and their control of tea-making facilities reflected their reward power over the doctors – the absence of a cup of tea during surgery often announcing their censure. The nursing staff – State Registered Nurses – regarded themselves as superior to receptionists because of the expert power related to professional status and this accentuated conflict in line management to the practice manager.

The concept of a Primary Care Team was not recognised and District Nurses, Midwives, etc., were not regarded as part of the organisation. However, the District Health Authority clinic was situated close to the surgery and its proximity facilitated communication, in part compensating for this deficiency.

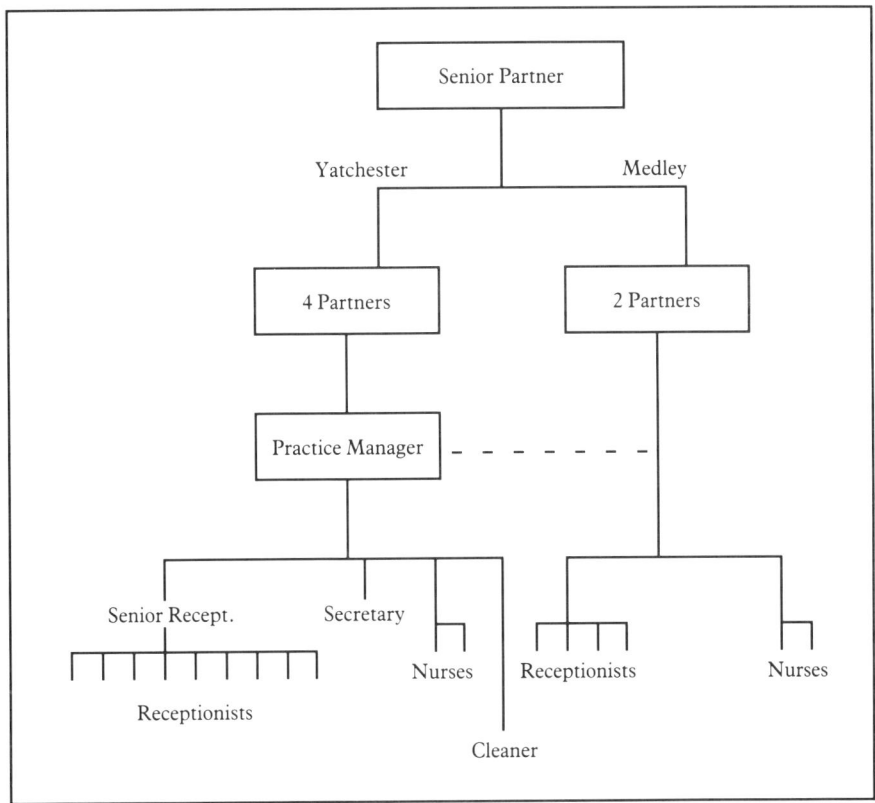

Diagram 2.25 The formal organisation of the Yatchester and Medley group practice

Process

Yatchester was, therefore, the traditional centre of 'power' in the practice, with the senior partner and majority of the partners at the administrative

127

base of the organisation, with constant support from the practice manager and secretary. The division of the partners into two teams resulted in a dominant coalition consisting of the Yatchester based doctors grouped around the senior partner. Practice policy was firmly controlled by them and proposals for change were easily resisted. The two systems developed their own characteristics and there was an increasing dichotomy of opinion and practice.

Patient care
Donabedian (1966) has suggested that quality of care to patients can be audited in three dimensions – structure, process and outcome (Diagram 2.26). Although it is not the remit of this critique to audit clinical decisions, it is evident that the structure and process elements reflect the practice organisation and that patient satisfaction is an outcome measure.

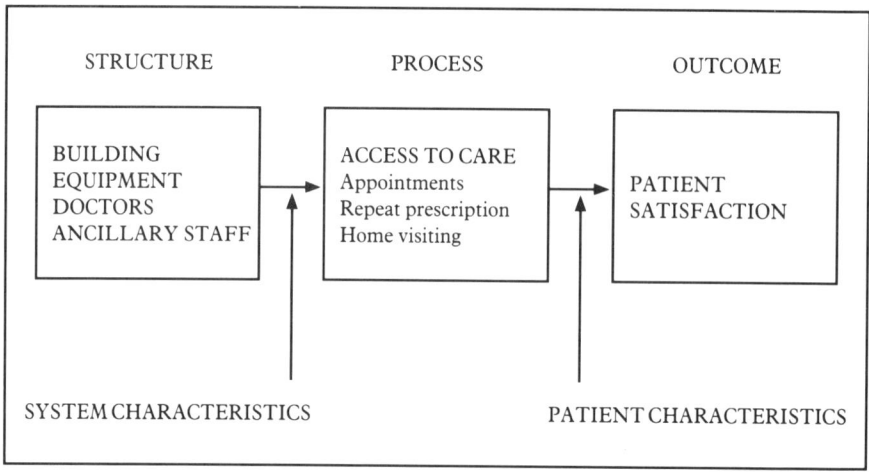

Diagram 2.26 Structure, process and outcome in General Practice

It will be obvious from the previous discussion that the surgery facilities in Yatchester were inadequate to cope with patient demands, restricting availability of appointments and increasing demand on emergency facilities, both in requests for home visits and the use of the emergency clinics. 'Emergencies' were seen at the end of the routine surgeries after screening by a nurse in the treatment room, and numbers on occasions exceeded booked appointments. A chronic shortage of appointments perpetuated this system and patients learned to bypass the 'system,' to obtain access to care, and the outcome was apparent:

Patient satisfaction was low.
Staff morale was low, due to stress and unpredictable hours.
Increased demand for domiciliary visits.

There was, however, a resistance to modify the system to compensate – among doctors, the philosophy prevailed that 'when you're working it's extremely busy but there's plenty of time off'. There was a reluctance to increase the length of consulting hours and, indeed, this was subject to finite limits due to the restricted accommodation.

The demands placed on reception staff were increased by a high demand for repeat prescriptions which was based on patients' records that were frequently unstructured. There was little attempt to summarise case notes and correspondence was frequently not filed in chronological order, merely being 'tucked into' the Lloyd George envelope. Limited secretarial support delayed preparation of referral letters for hospital care.

The doctor:patient ratio placed the practice in the 'designated area' (underdoctored) category. There was a resistance to increase the number of partners in the practice in spite of this, partly due to the physical constraints of the building, but also because of the potential financial implications. To some degree, the allowances payable to Designated Areas – although intended by Government to increase recruitment – in fact had the reverse effect! As a result of the high demand for care and the inability of the system to cope, patient complaints increased and the morale of staff deteriorated.

Administration
The senior partner had traditionally dominated the organisation and controlled dealings with the accountant, practice bankers and the Family Practitioner Committee (FPC) – delegation was rare. Except on major issues – such as replacement of a partner – formal meetings were infrequent, and often convened only in response to a crisis. Administrative decisions were often autonomous or made following a 'straw poll', usually amongst the practitioners at Yatchester – the dominant coalition. Despite this criticism, the majority of partners consented to this pattern of administration. The practice manager had little managerial autonomy and had a reactive role coordinating duty rotas and dealing with staffing issues. She was responsible for collating and submitting claims for fees and allowances to the FPC, but otherwise had no role in the financial affairs and was excluded from practice meetings.

The business affairs of the practice were relatively unstructured and despite the size of the financial turnover, equating to that of a small firm, accountancy methods were primitive. Personnel issues never featured high on agendas and relied on the implicit loyalty of staff who were almost all patients of the practice. Despite the variable duration of surgeries, staff rarely received overtime payments, rates of pay being negotiated locally. This latter hurdle was overcome in the early 1980s, when the more enlightened partners were able to negotiate acceptance of the Whitley Council recommendations in the face of staff unrest – a major plank of the argument being that the FPC reimbursed 70% of ancillary staff wages under the terms of the Statement of Fees and Allowances (*Red Book*).

Conclusions

This brief critique reveals that the organisation had not adapted to demand, and that its apparent complacency reflected the absence of clear goals, enshrined in any kind of mission statement, for the development of the practice. Its primary task was maintenance of the status quo with maximisation of income at the least effort. This survival task reflected the lack of vision of the partners, who seemed complacent about the changes imminent in primary care and the need to pay greater attention to the consumers and their views. The building in the High Street had outlived its usefulness and the need for alternative accommodation was critical to the future of the practice. The fabric of the premises and facilities available probably represented the minimum standards acceptable to the Family Practitioner Committee. As a consequence, financial sanction was a possibility, as reimbursement of notional rent and rates was dependent upon the Committee being satisfied with surgery premises.

'The time is ripe, and rotten ripe, for change; Then let it come.'

Lowell
A Glance Behind the Curtain

Negotiation for change

From the article so far, it is probably obvious that I have identified the need for change, and also that I was based at the branch surgery at Medley. Another young colleague in Medley, Dr Brown and I had detected the symptoms of decay and had discussed the options available. Briefly, these were to:

a. influence change by expanding the partnership, developing new premises, and the revision of current practice organisation;
b. seek to dissolve the partnership and establish Medley as a separate practice unit; or
c. resign from the practice.

In assessing the merits of these options, it became obvious that it would be difficult to separate Medley from the mainsteam practice because of restrictive clauses in the partnership agreement and the likelihood that the remaining partners would not consent to the move. In addition, the logistics of arranging a two-man practice proved to be a barrier for Dr Brown. Resignation became an option if we were unsuccessful in

influencing change. Tentative discussions with the remaining partners confirmed our estimates of the resistance expected, which reflected:
– a lack of perceived need for change
– a reluctance to consider change during final years in practice – three of the partners nearing planned retirement at the age of 60 years
– a reluctance to accept financial risk.

At this stage we defined the following characteristics of the organisation:

Yatchester
Strengths: Traditional centre of 'power'.
                  Administrative base of the practice.
                  Base for the majority of partners.
                  Consulting hours – open 11 sessions per week.
                  Base for the Practice Manager.

Weaknesses: Relative unresponsiveness to patient demand.
                  Shortage of appointments.
                  High demand for repeat prescriptions.
                  Poor staff morale.
                  Inadequate premises.
                  Lack of goals and a mission statement.

Medley
Strengths: Purpose built health centre (Local Authority).
                  Staff morale high.
                  More responsive to patient demand.
                  Prescription monitoring policy in operation.
                  Defined goals and mission statement.
                  A cohesive alliance between partners.
                  Patient loyalty and a strong village identity.

Weaknesses: Restricted consulting hours – 9 sessions a week.
                  Isolation from the dominant coalition/powerbase.
                  Vulnerability of a 'two-man' lobby – labelling as 'Young Turks'.
                  Minimal input from Practice Manager.

Our defined Mission Statement was:
1. To obtain modern surgery premises in Yatchester, to enable
2. expansion of partnership size, to enable
3. provision of an expanded range of patient services which would be responsive to demand.
4. to review available computer systems to augment practice administrative and patient care.

Forster and Hadley, 1989, drawing on the work of Lewin, 1947; Dalton et al, 1968 and others, defined three factors in introducing change:
1. The weight of the countervailing forces favouring change and those resisting it.
2. The strategy developed to unfreeze resistance to change.
3. The dynamics of implementing the changes themselves.
Diagram 2.27 applies this approach to the situation in the practice.

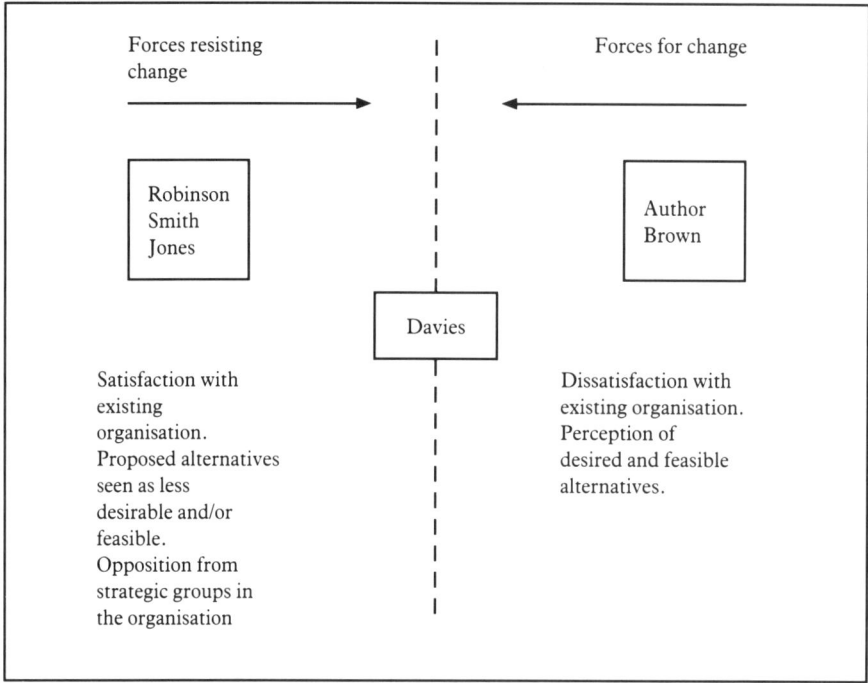

Diagram 2.27   Countervailing forces for and against change
in the Yatchester and Medley General Practice

The senior three partners, all nearing retirement, were understandably more resistant to change, whilst Dr Davies, of a similar age to ourselves, was known to be ambivalent. We determined during informal discussions that he supported much of the initiative but was concerned at the financial liabilities of the project. If that risk could be minimised, it seemed likely that he would support the proposals and the equation of power would be more favourably balanced. Financial considerations were also identified as a key demotivator of the senior partners, who were understandably reluctant to commit capital to the project and resisted erosion of their income.

Strategy

Success of the project seemed to be reliant upon a detailed and thorough presentation of the case based on careful research. We sought advice from local colleagues who had built their own surgeries, determining the planning process, and the methods of finance. Visits to the premises revealed design features that could be incorporated in our own project and highlighted problems to be avoided. The Statement of Fees and Allowances (*Red Book*), which defined the standards of accommodation, was studied carefully, as this also had a bearing on the financial arrangements. In addition, information was collected on the workload – numbers of appointments, visits, repeat prescriptions and waiting times – at both surgery sites, demonstrating the current deficiencies.

Previous informal attempts to introduce change were blighted because of the inadequate preparation and the lack of availability of documentation at the meetings. On this occasion, a project briefing document was to be prepared for presentation to the partners. In the interim, opportunities were taken to 'lobby' individual partners on the deficiencies of the present system and the benefits to be accrued from change.

Dynamics of change

Early in 1985, the case for a new building and expansion of the partnership was outlined at the annual holiday meeting, when the mood was affable. It was agreed to consider the proposal at a future meeting when further information was to be presented. The case then relied on our extensive research and a succinct presentation which pre-empted many of the likely questions. In particular:

Financial issues
- capital payments would not fall due until the building was complete;
- the cost-rent scheme effectively gave an interest-free loan provided that criteria in the Statement of Fees and Allowances were met;
- the impact of taking an additional partner would be balanced by the additional allowances gained and the increase in fees for items of service;
- as a neighbouring practice was about to take an extra partner, the designated area allowance for under-doctored areas would be lost anyway.

Management issues
- the project timetable enabled change to be incremental;
- enabled introduction of additional services, eg a diabetes clinic;
- reduction of individual workload;
- pre-empting the likely intervention of the FPC;
- facilitated future developments including a possible move to training practice status with financial benefits.

In the event, the proposals were favourably received and, following lengthy debate of the financial issues, it was agreed to discuss the project with the FPC and the Regional Medical Officer. The senior partner was allowed to lead this initiative and the sense of ownership that he developed increased his enthusiasm. Discussions with the practice solicitor enabled us to develop the partnership agreement to incorporate clauses protecting the interests of retiring partners, preventing any potential loss on any capital invested.

Having demonstrated our capacity and willingness to manage the project, the partners were content to devolve lead responsibilities. It was agreed that Dr Brown would accept responsibility for the financial aspects and that I would coordinate project management. Whilst this relieved the 'elder statesmen' of the burden, the delegation of management transferred control to the 'Young Turks', making an important change in the practice dynamics.

The building project could form a lengthy study in its own right, but the next section identifies some of the features which are pertinent to the evolution of the practice and its eventual destabilisation.

The new surgery

The availability of suitable sites was restricted and we had to consider patient access and the availability of existing pharmaceutical services. Fortunately our project coincided with the redevelopment of the town centre and our application was dealt with very sympathetically by the local planning authority. Initial financial arrangements were made with the General Practice Finance Corporation (a government agency) but, on the day our formal application was submitted, a moratorium of lending was imposed as a result of a change in government policy.

Subsequent financial arrangements with a bank gained both better interest rates and a deferrment of capital repayment, further alleviating any burden on retiring partners.

Destabilisation

In addition to the demands and pressures generated by a major building project and practice reorganisation, the practice also faced other formidable challenges. Doctors Smith and Jones both retired prematurely due to ill health during the project, necessitating recruitment of two new partners. The practice manager tendered her resignation to be effective at the time of transfer to the new surgery in August, 1988 and the practice, therefore, had to recruit a practice manager at a time of critical change. To compound events, during preparations for the official opening of the surgery, I was admitted to the local coronary care unit. As a direct consequence, Dr Brown decided that the personal burdens and sacrifices were too great and resigned early in 1988, to take up another post. This was a severe blow, as the loss of a key member of the management team at a critical time of practice development increased the process of destabilisation.

The NHS changes increased the demands on primary care and associated with the burden of 'out of hours' work, led to Dr Davies' resignation in the autumn of 1988, to take up a non-clinical post. With a planned retirement early in 1990, Dr Robinson, the senior partner, was the only person declaring optimism in the face of the introduction of the GP Contract on 1st April, 1990. In the spring of 1990, I succeeded Dr Robinson as senior partner but ironically on the same day, accepted an appointment in elsewhere and subsequently tendered my resignation to the practice.

The outcome

In conclusion, it is perhaps reasonable to assess the outcome and balance the gains against the losses.

Gains

Modern Surgery Premises
– spacious accommodation
– 5 consulting suites
– fully equipped treatment room
– adequate administrative areas
– modern records system
– accommodation for ancillary staff
Computerisation
Increase to 7 partners
Expanded appointment time
Expanded range of services
– clinics, minor surgery

Hospital consultants providing
    out-patient clinics on site
Regular practice meetings
Recruitment of a progressive
    practice manager
Structured case notes
Improved secretarial support
A business filing system
Enhanced financial
    management
A corporate image

Losses

Staff
The staff complained of the increased workload and extended surgery hours in the new system and found that it took longer to service consulting suites which were more widely dispersed.
The spaciousness of the building resulted in reduced contact with other staff.
New working practices introduced by a new practice manager initially increased tension.

Partners
The demands of the GP Contract and extended surgery hours led to complaints regarding increased workload.

New working practices and an increase in partnership size resulted in a change of longstanding rotas.

Practice meetings, held on a regular monthly basis, generated demands for a more rapid pace of change despite the instability of the system. This generated tension and acrimony and the formation of new alliances.

The role of the senior partner had been eroded and the power base of the practice became destabilised.

Epilogue

I left the practice in the summer of 1990, since when there have been further changes in partnership and an increase to eight partners.

With the advantage of hindsight it is clear that the change was planned with technical and financial matters uppermost in our minds. On such criteria it could reasonably be said to have been a success. However, in terms of human relationships it was profoundly destabilising to the point, in fact, where it has been extremely difficult to establish a new equilibrium over the succeeding years. Retrospectively, it can be seen that the conditions in which the changes were negotiated and launched did not encourage open discussion and exploration of the possible consequences of the reorganisation for social relationships within the practice.

The dominant coalition was initially reluctant to agree to the changes and was only persuaded to accept them when the material advantages became clear and on the understanding that the hard work involved in planning all the details would be taken on by the 'Young Turks' from Medley. In this process, the human factors in change were simply sidelined. When these factors made themselves felt, no one was prepared and the viability of the team was clearly at risk.

How far the failure to work through and try to compensate for the strains and stresses of the reorganisation contributed to the illness, early retirement, and resignations that accompanied the reorganisation is impossible to determine. The major changes that were going on in the NHS as a whole at the same time also certainly had their impact. What is evident, however, is that the new negotiated order was not sufficiently strong or stable to absorb the consequences of the changed situation. New doctors had to be recruited rapidly to the practice. There was little time or inclination to engage in team-building strategies. Dalton et al's (1968) conditions for the successful implementation of change including the development of specific goals, heightened self-esteem, and internalising the motives for change did not seem to be present. Organisational drift rather than sense of direction characterised the management of the practice.

'Whoever thinks a faultless piece to see,
thinks what ne'er was, nor is, nor e'er shall be'

Pope, *Essay on Criticism*,
lines 253, 254.

Case Study 10: Change in a rural General Practice

A General Practitioner

Editors' introduction
The general practice which provides the focus for this study had seen little development or change over a long period of time. The author notes this initially as a paradox but subsequently unravels some of the personal and local reasons for the lack of development. In the context of the national picture of general practice, the running of the practice prior to the arrival of the author was indeed somewhat anachronistic. General practice as a profession had been through a period of conflict with the government much earlier in the 1960s to achieve financial backing for many of the changes subsequently perceived to be beneficial to this particular practice. The charter for general practice, agreed in 1965, arose out of general practitioners' dissatisfaction with their status, pay and conditions of work by comparison with those of hospital consultants (Fry, 1988). The charter introduced a remuneration package which, amongst other effects, favoured group practice and especially team work through the direct reimbursement of 70 per cent of the cost of employing ancillary staff.

This Case Study also exemplifies how progressive general practice embraces a holistic view of the individual patient. In the circumstances of this study, this is represented by a wish to provide care and counselling for problems beyond those purely medical or physical in origin and consequently has to take into account the influences and background of each patient's life. This holistic view of the individual is echoed by a similar approach to the organisation (the practice) that will be required to deliver this style of care. The author, therefore, describes for the reader not only the internal dynamics of this small organisation but the external forces to which it was responding, for example the concern of the DHA and FHSA about the 'performance indicators' for the practice.

Organisational perspectives: the author makes very effective use of a wide range of analytical tools to explore his subject but this study is particularly interesting as an example of an attempt to deploy a blend of consultative and participative management styles (Introduction, pages 26–7) in the introduction of change. This approach appears highly successful, but falters at the point where the author, who is also the principal actor, is temporarily removed from the scene by sick leave, and is replaced by his newly recruited partner who prefers a more traditional style of management. The end result, on the return of the author, was the negotiation of a compromise between their two approaches. We are left to choose between two alternative lessons which might be drawn from this story and which are considered by the author: was this retrenchment the result of his choice of the wrong partner, resulting from failure to carry the principles of participative management to their logical conclusion and share the appointing process fully with his team? Or was it an inevitable development, once the first heady years of developing the new practice were over, and a more robust and less personal model of management was required?

The Case Study

In this Case Study I describe a series of changes in a small rural practice during a five year period. I start with a simple description of the facts regarding the practice up to the study period. I then take a systems approach to discuss briefly the nature of general practice, possible alternative models of practice types, and specifically to define the model into which I attempted to change the practice in question: that of the primary health care team. I describe my objectives for change and the plan that was used to attempt to bring about the change. I then use more of an action perspective to describe what actually happened, concentrating on aspects of the plan which worked well, the negotiated position by the end of the time period, and an evaluation of that position. In conclusion I will attempt to explain why it appears, with reference to the original objectives, that some things went wrong, although the end result was a success.

Introduction

> 'The best laid schemes of mice and men gang aft a-gley'
>
> Robert Burns

Two doctors, *Dr A* and *Dr B*, left national service just in time to join the new National Health Service (NHS) in 1948. They purchased what had been a small single-handed rural practice and set about expanding it. In the early 1950s they moved out of the 'back kitchen' of one of the doctor's homes into a purpose built surgery at the bottom of the other doctor's garden. They were justifiably proud of what was then an innovatory move.

General Practice was very much the Cinderella of the NHS, which in the 1950s could almost have been called the National Hospital Service. General Practitioners (GPs) had a low status, with relatively small reward; they tended to work individually and without any structured support from other professions (like district nurses). But these two GPs were farsighted enough to invest in premises and attract sufficient patients from a wide area to make the practice reasonably successful. It is therefore an unexplained paradox that no further development took place. From 1952 until the start of the study period very little changed. The practice was administered by the GPs themselves, with the help of only their wives. The premises remained untouched. The prescribing practices (the GPs dispensed medicines to all their patients, there was no chemist in the area) remained archaic. No written records were kept, very few regular claims or administrative returns were made, consultation times and methods were fossilised and many old-fashioned surgical and obstetric practices were maintained and carried out with almost reckless disregard for modern methods.

It is hardly an exaggeration to describe the practice as a cross between *Dr Finlay* and *The Citadel*. A.J. Cronin could have created it! The dispensary was stocked with drugs that dated back to the 1920s. Re-usable needles and glass syringes were being used. 'Kitchen table' surgery was being practised. Midwifery remained the domain of the GPs, who were still carrying out operative deliveries at home. Chloroform was still in use as an anaesthetic. Modern treatments were sometimes unknown. Certain non-fatal conditions were still being treated as 'terminal'. There were only open surgeries; held each day at 9am and 6pm (including Saturdays). Huge numbers of home visits were carried out. Magic and humbug were in regular use: 'You have sent for me just in time; I'll see what I can do to save you!' (for a mild problem!).

At the beginning of the study period, a few months before *Dr B* planned to retire, *Dr A* died. It is worth noting that *Dr A* had always been the 'senior partner', because of age rather than length of time in the practice. He had delegated no responsibility for the financial affairs of the practice, and appeared to have been the leader in almost all of the decisions, few that they were, that the partnership made. When he died, the administration of the practice, the filing system, records, protocols and methods died with him. *Dr B* was a kind, gentle and sincerely motivated GP. He recognised that he was old fashioned but he was happy with the role he had played for 35 years in his partner's shadow. He was increasingly concerned with his garden and his hobbies and was looking forward to retirement. His wife was reluctant to remain tied to the practice (the only telephone was at *Dr A*'s house, for example) and was looking forward to her husband's retirement with even greater relish. I arrived into a situation which could almost be described as the proverbial 'green-field' site. As an organisation, the practice was almost completely nonexistent. The patients were still there, *Dr B* was willing to continue in a part-time capacity for a short period, there was no effective competition and the Family Practitioner Committee and District Health Authority were keen to see improvements. It was therefore possible for me to attempt to choose the best option and bring about the changes that I felt were the most desirable to develop the practice and bring it into the modern era.

A systems analysis of General Practice:

'But I was thinking of a plan
To dye one's whiskers green.'

Lewis Carroll

As an organisation, what is the mission of general practice? Most health-related organisations, when they attempt to define their mission, come to state rather platitudinous and or altruistic ideas about helping people, and GPs would be no different. They would probably agree to a formula which gave prominence to the aims of improving the quality and quantity of people's lives. It is important to recognise that, in the United Kingdom, GPs are independent contractors who run their own small businesses. They generally contract most of their time to the NHS but they remain responsible for the running of their business, the maintenance of their premises, payment of their expenses, staff salaries and so forth. They therefore have a clear and unambiguous survival goal or primary purpose. This can be defined as aiming to satisfy enough people, to keep the practice list large enough, to attract sufficient fees to pay all of the bills and make enough profit to pay the partners according to their expectations.

There is a partial explanation here for the state of affairs when I arrived. The two GPs were satisfied with their income and saw no reason to change; I would not have been satisfied in the long term – because of what was available to me elsewhere – and saw change as the only viable route to a higher income. An honest appraisal of the primary purpose puts some aspects of motivation in context!

Systems thinking emerges from two main strands of thought and its emergence and usefulness in organisational theory dates back to the 1930s and 1940s. Aristotle had seen that a whole was more than the sum of its parts; but modern science from the seventeenth century onwards had tended to disregard his view of the world. By the beginning of this century science had itself become so complex and subdivided that it was difficult to understand what was happening or how things worked. Engineering, for instance, was quintessentially involved in making things work; particularly in electrical engineering and communications. Biologists, meanwhile, maintained their 'organic' view of the way things were, and it was a biologist who brought these two philosophies together and gave them a more generalised footing – systems thinking (von Bertalanffy, 1950).

Organisations are describable in terms of an open system. There is a balance between what goes into the system and what comes out. The system is responsible for the transformation of these inputs into outputs. For most systems, many subsystems can be described that support the process. General Practice appears to me to be a system that takes money and patients (who are anxious, poorly, dependent, and so on) and transforms these inputs into patients who are now confident, satisfied, well, independent, etc., and into a 'reputation'. The quality of these outputs feeds back, via the community in which the practice operates, to attract more patients and more money into the system. Diagram 2.28 illustrates this system. Furthermore, when one considers the flow of patients, General Practice is one of a number of other systems sharing a similar mission. For example, hospitals, social services, community health authority staff such as district nurses and health visitors, and voluntary groups might all define their goals in a similar way.

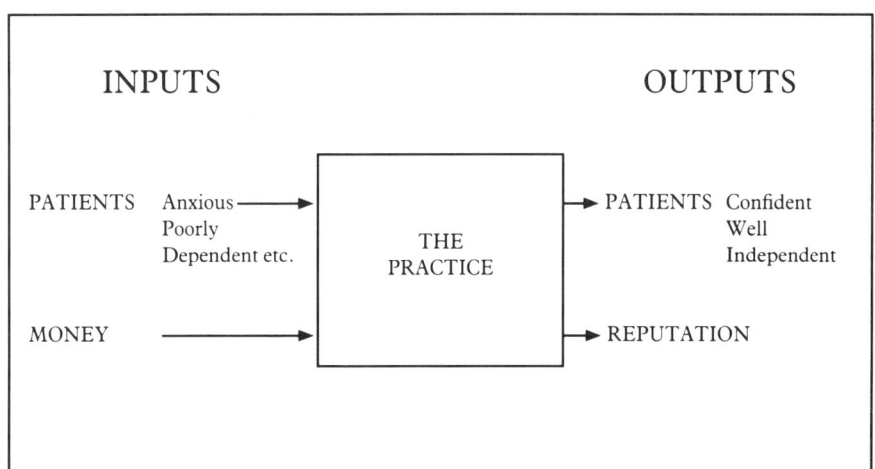

Diagram 2.28   General Practice as an 'open system'

Using the model shown in Diagram 2.29, it is possible to identify some characteristics of the system run by the original doctors:
– Shared mission. They were attempting the same overall task as any other GPs, and other similar organisations in the area.

– Neglect of the primary purpose. By the time *Dr A* died the list size was falling and their accounts revealed a falling income.

– Restriction of 'inputs'. Their model of practice was limited to a very strict definition of the 'patient'. They did not operate a system designed to cope with emotional distress, mild self-limiting illness, inadequacy or moral feebleness (by their definitions). Their system had no 'pastoral' function and patients had to have recognisable medical illness, preferably severe, to gain access.

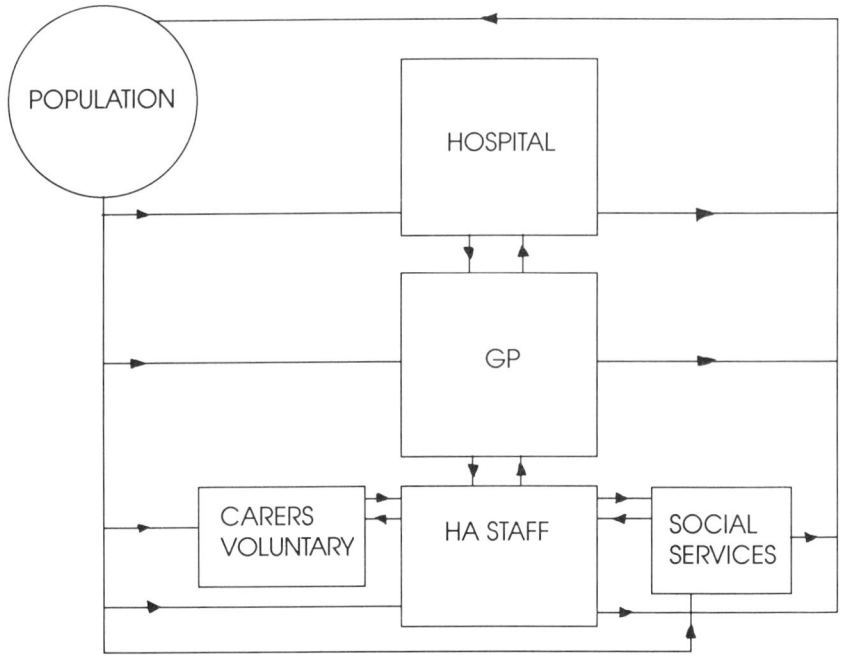

Diagram 2.29   The flow of patients between systems with a shared mission

– Disregard of 'outputs'. Their model relied upon conservatism amongst their patients rather than obvious success in problem solving or reliance on reputation to feedback and attract more 'business'.

– Independence. Their system was not in contact with any other neighbouring system sharing the same mission. They maintained very clear boundaries and kept the hospital, district nurses, etc., at a considerable distance.

The primary health care team

> This very remarkable man
> Commends a most practical plan

You can do what you want
If you don't think you can't
So don't think you can't if you can

Charles Inge

These systems that share a common mission can be made to work as sub-systems of a single unit which we call the Primary Health Care Team (PHCT), illustrated by Diagram 2.30. My training, background and immediate needs (for example, to relieve my wife of being tied to the telephone by employing a receptionist) led me to believe the PHCT was a more appropriate model. Its characteristics were to be:

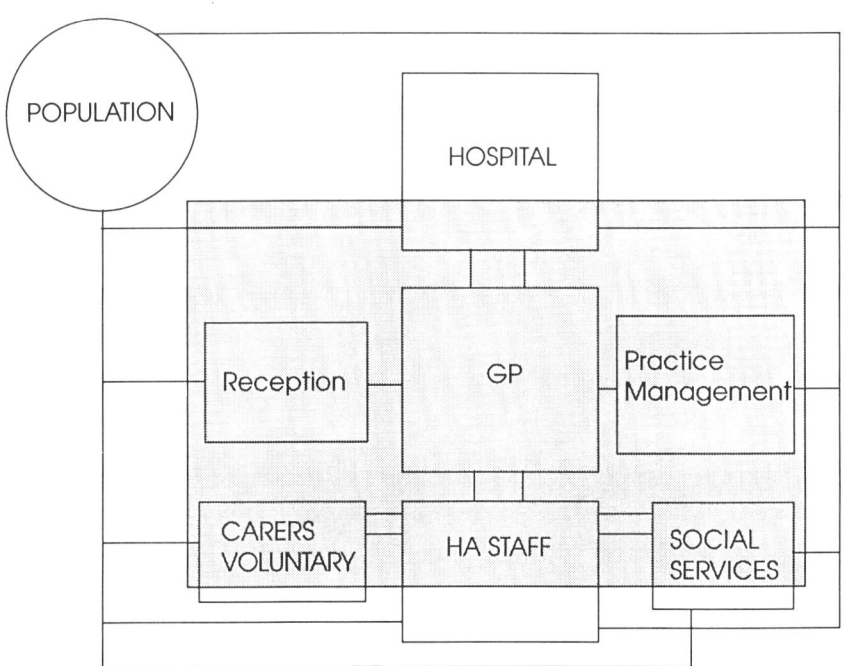

Diagram 2.30   The primary health care team

– Adherence to the mission and the primary purpose. Altruism and platitudes were not enough. The quality of care was a very desirable ultimate goal but the practice also had to make more money.
– Broadened and increased inputs. Patients would be allowed, and wherever possible encouraged, to enter the system according to their own definition of need.
– Re-drawn system boundaries. Health visitors, district nurses and midwives, social workers, lay carers, hospital consultants, etc., would

now all be part of the system. Teamwork, appropriate delegation and the maximum use of expertise, in job roles carrying high degrees of discretion, would be the norm.

– New subsystems. Reception and managerial staff would be employed and deployed to maintain the system, to improve communications within the system, etc.

– A new infrastructure. The practice needed new premises.

In sum, the new model was so radically different that a lot of change was required. Having decided on such a model, my two main objectives were to manage the change as sensitively as possible, and to build in some evaluation to ensure it was all worthwhile.

The process of change

'I can resist everything except temptation'

Oscar Wilde

Why had the situation in this practice remained so 'stuck' in a particular model? By the last years of the old practice, there were a number of interested parties wanting to see change: *Dr B* was well aware he and *Dr A* had 'let things go'. He had a lot of professional guilt about the standards, the state of the records and so on. Now close to retirement, he wanted to leave on a 'higher note' and counteract the significant danger that his practice would disappear.

– The District Health Authority (DHA) was very unhappy about records not being kept. The practice was bottom of the district league for vaccination uptake.

– The Family Practitioner Committee (FPC) – now Family Health Services Authority (FHSA) – was equally disturbed about the state of the services, the premises and the records. They had had to deal with a number of complaints about the practice and were threatening to withdraw certain allowances (notional rent, for example) if things didn't change.

– The local population were voting with their feet. They were having to put up with a number of inefficient practices (no appointments, for example) and the practice list was falling.

– The community staff were suffering from lack of cooperation and real communication. Appropriate tasks were not being delegated and they were given no discretion.

– Local professionals. Other GPs and local hospital consultants were expressing concern about standards.

These examples of the shared dissatisfaction with the practice at this time seem to be overwhelming, yet nothing was happening! Change can only occur if the sum of these factors can overcome the resistance to change. *Doctors A and B* were extremely conservative. Their habits and methods had changed little since the early 1950s and they were comfortable with their style. The local population was ultimately responsible. The majority accepted the status quo. In this rural area they were also sufficiently parochial not to know what they were missing. It tended to be newcomers who complained or joined other (town) practices. They did not share the same expectations of a good doctor. Because the practice satisfied many local people, it did not change. There was, in effect, a balance between the forces of dissatisfaction and the resistance to change. When I arrived, initially I joined both sides, wanting to see change and create my own model of good practice (the PHCT), yet being at first reluctant to take on the challenge because of the anticipated work and personal cost (see Diagram 2.31).

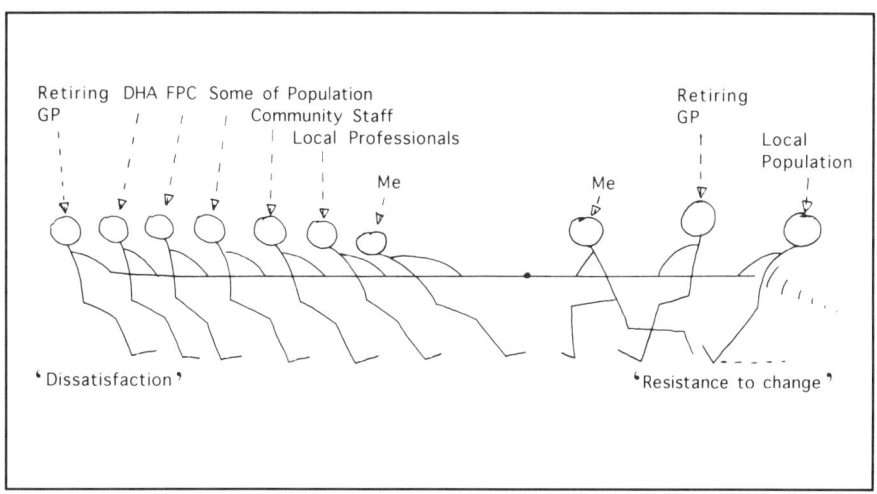

Diagram 2.31   The change 'tug of war'

Using the model described by Forster and Hadley (1989), I now recognise two phases in the changes I subsequently led:
Firstly, change became inevitable. The sum of the dissatisfaction with the existing organisation, the clear vision I had of an alternative and the backing for change coming from the FPC (who would provide, amongst other things, money to invest in the new practice) overwhelmed any resistance or opposition.
Secondly, my goals and motives were shared by many other players. I was particularly fortunate with the people who joined in the process of change. The District Nurse/Midwife, the Health Visitor and the first few members of staff I employed all became very important to the success of the venture. The strategy then, of moving to the general goal of a

functioning PHCT, involved planning a series of specific goals that incorporated the ideas of these other people, heightened their self-esteem and used their support to fix, or 're-freeze', the new model. Apart from people, the other key elements in the strategy were the coherent integration of their efforts and the provision of a proper home for the practice.

Team building and system evolution

The Receptionist. Georgia was our next door neighbour when we first moved to the village. She was bright and had had a lot of office experience before marrying a local man. She had not worked since having her children and, apart from a little book work for her husband, was not using her skills at all. She had exactly the right kind of careful, almost obsessional personality to take on the practice administration. She single-handedly created files and records for the 2,000 patients, and card-index systems for an age-sex register which was subsequently developed and used for vaccination administration, and cervical smear recalls. She saw in the development of changed surgery hours, appointment systems, new dispensing arrangements and many other aspects of patient orientated administration. She also quickly learned (either from me or the courses she went on!) the relationship of the practice (as a small business) with the FPC, and no more claims were ever forgotten or missed. She rapidly changed her own role from part-time receptionist to indispensable practice manager.

The District Nurse. Although close to retirement herself, Virginia appeared to have been waiting all of her life for the opportunity to develop her own ideas. Together we completely realigned the focus of domiciliary care (from GP to Nurse) and she carried out virtually all the necessary assessments and care plans for patients needing home visits. She took on all the treatment policy decisions for incontinence, bed-sores, stroke rehabilitation and terminal care. We set up and jointly ran a cervical smear/well woman clinic and in her role as District Midwife she started an ante-natal service which rapidly took over from the hospital-based service which mothers had had to accept previously.

The Health Visitor. Less of a charismatic personality, perhaps, but nonetheless an innovator, Caroline also relished the opportunities presented by increased discretion in her role. In less than three years, we transformed our standing in the 'vaccination league' from bottom to top of the DHA list. Caroline ran her own child surveillance clinic and was instrumental in our starting an elderly surveillance system (long before the government thought of putting it in the GP contract).

The Practice Nurse. In an attempt to meet some of the need for woman to woman consultations, I employed a nurse to operate as an independent practitioner within the team. Louise ran her own surgeries and developed her own style alongside the things we were able to do together – like a diabetic clinic, for example.

All of the specific projects detailed above were part of a strategy to integrate the team. I tried to use their ideas as much as possible. We ran a continuous Practice meeting every morning at coffee time and everyone was welcome. Other team members, like the community psychiatric nurse, the social worker and the 'bath nurse' had equal access and enjoyed the atmosphere of shared objectives and motives.

During this time we planned, designed and built new premises with good treatment, office, staff and waiting facilities to replace the rudimentary building of the old practice. The rebuilding was financed using the so-called 'cost-rent' scheme. GPs mostly own their own practice premises. When they make approved changes to these premises or build entirely new ones, they have the option of taking the reimbursement which they get for renting their premises to the NHS in the form of 'cost-rent'. This figure is based on the capital cost of the new premises, and is approximately equal to the cost of borrowing the capital to carry out the building project. This effectively means that GPs can take out a mortgage on new premises and that the entire cost is reimbursed! An interest free loan! It is a good and popular scheme and goes a long way to explain why most GPs work in really good premises. In my practice we were able to carry out a £88,000 rebuilding programme which, because it was also eligible for an improvement grant, and because the banks regard GPs as such good risks, we were able to raise the capital at only fractionally above the base rate, and ended up creating a net increase in practice income.

I saw myself as very much what McGregor has described as a 'Theory Y' manager (McGregor, 1960). In other words, I believed that people's commitment to their jobs will be greatest where their work satisfies significant elements of their own needs; that if people share the goals of the organisation they do not need close supervision to make them work; and that in the right conditions, people can learn to seek and accept responsibility. I believed that previously the people involved in the work of the practice had been seriously underused. By the process of unlimited delegation and the encouragement of high levels of discretion in their activities everyone was very happy and committed to seeing the PHCT work. Certainly, we were committed to the objectives, and derived a lot of pleasure and fulfilment from the work, not the least of which was the increased satisfaction of the patients with the practice. The strengths of the system were now revealed. The practice prospered and expanded. Despite the hugely increased practice expenses (staff, buildings, etc.) the profit rose handsomely. The service we were offering, with reference to the mission task, was undeniably improved.

The weaknesses of the system were also revealed. The team worked so well it was a little self-indulgent. Outsiders found it difficult to work with us, and occasional changes in personnel were difficult. (One new part-time receptionist for example, lasted only one month). The high discretion in certain roles (for example, the practice nurse) depended very heavily on mutual trust. The cosiness of the original team also depended to some extent on the shared horror of the old system. As things became more normal, and particularly when we moved into the new premises, the commitment to change was obviously diluted.

Most of these changes took three years to implement. *Dr B* had by then completely retired and the increasing size of the practice made a new full-time partner possible. He was just about to start when I unfortunately had to spend seven months on sick leave. By the time I returned to work, and during the following six months or so, the system changed again. On this occasion, the changes were not brought about so much as a result of planning as the end result of negotiations between myself and the new partner, the new partner and the other team members.

The negotiated order

> 'The good old rule
> Sufficeth them, the simple plan,
> That they should take, who have the power,
> And they should keep who can.'
>
> William Wordsworth

To summarise the situation after three years, an organisation had come into being (almost from nothing) with the following characteristics:

It was an open system, taking patients and money, transforming them into well people and 'reputation'.

The 'dominant coalition' was a successful team sharing the same mission (improving quality and quantity of life for the client) and working to the same primary purpose (earning money).

I was leading the team as a result of my contract with the FPC. The ultimate clinical responsibility was mine and therefore I was granted the casting vote in decision taking.

The team was, however, run as a democratic, 'organic' collective. I saw my role totally as a *Theory Y* manager in a participative organisation. Likert has decribed such organisations in his classification of leadership styles as System 4 and shown how relationships within them are more appropriately represented by overlapping areas of responsibility than by traditional hierarchies (Likert, 1967). Diagram 2.32 shows how I conceptualised the practice organisation at the time.

The structure of the team was therefore characterised by few rules and little obvious hierarchy. Individual roles were indistinctly defined and all the jobs carried high levels of discretion. Mistakes were managed as

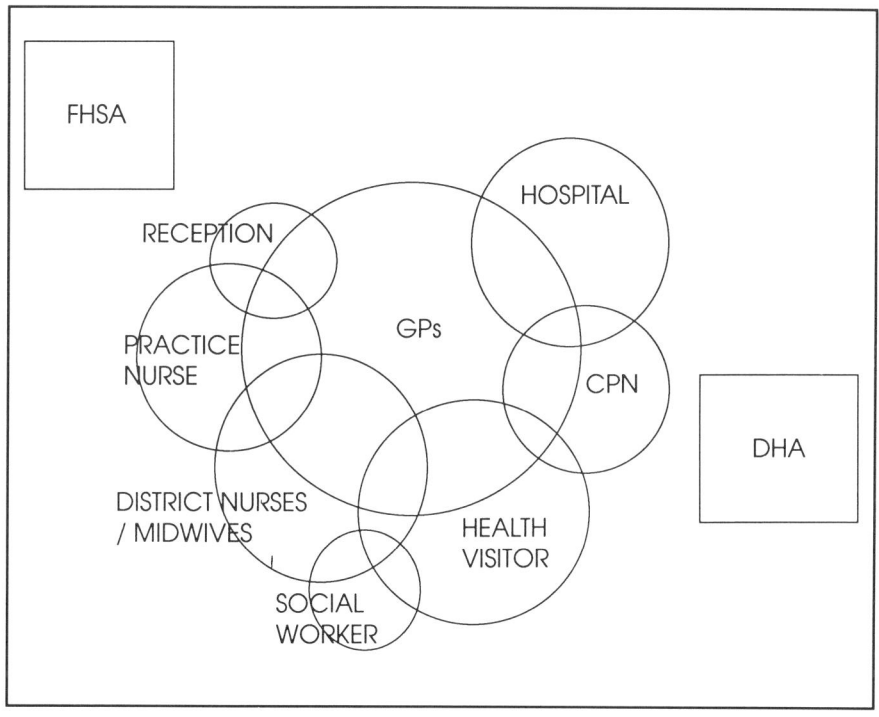

Diagram 2.32   The system 4 picture

educational experiences and training was shared, each according to needs and skill.

Expert power was the only overt authority used. Each team member had control of the decisions in their domain.

As I have said, the team thus became very cohesive. Although my leaving it for a period of seven months was outside my control, some of the team members felt subsequently 'betrayed'. My new partner, Washington, had not expected to find himself working with the team on his own – and worse – with a series of locums. His view of the way an organisation should work slowly emerged and proved to be somewhat different from the shared expectations of the PHCT. Washington's view was characterised by:

A bit more *Theory X*. Probably because he didn't know them, he was less sure that team members could be trusted. He tended to expect things to be done only if he directed it.

Efficient organisations require benevolent-authoritative (Likert's System 2), rather than participative leadership. Although benevolent, an organisation needed a defined structure and hierarchy (with, by implication, himself near the top). Diagram 2.33 shows his view of the desirable organisation for the practice team.

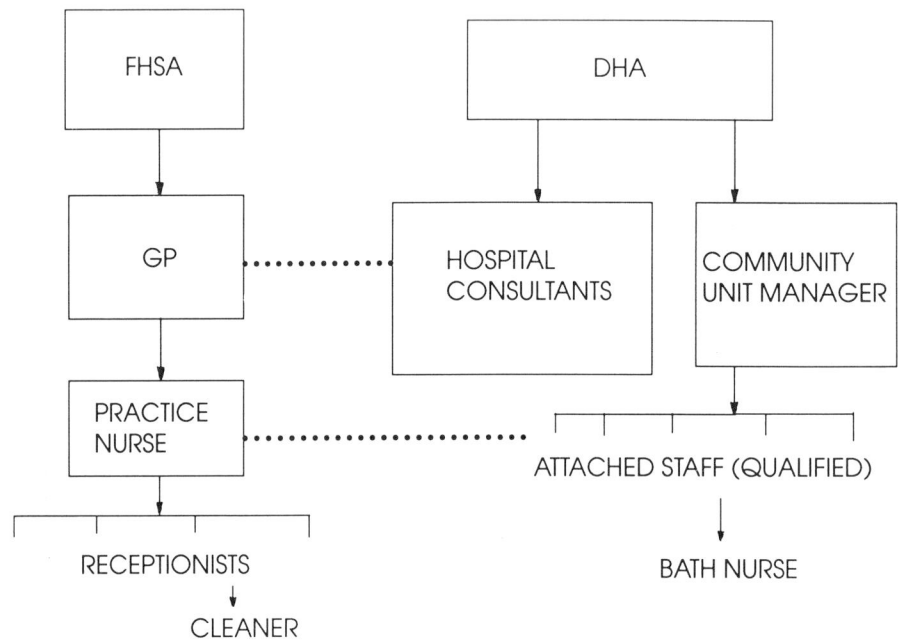

Diagram 2.33 Washington's view of the team

Safety and efficiency required more rules, protocols and so on.

Team meetings should be more formal and structured.

It is important to realise that he would not argue with the systems definition of the practice. In the appreciation of the mission and primary purpose, in the design of the subsystems and in the concept of a PHCT we were all completely agreed. He also agreed with the concept as the most efficient way of transforming our inputs into outputs. However, the differences between the visions of the organisation were clearly a source of potential conflict. After he assumed charge of the practice, changes immediately began to occur. The Practice Nurse resigned. The District Nurse took her retirement, sooner rather than later. Some reception staff changes took place. Understanding theories such as those about participative management is not enough as is clearly shown by the 'action perspective'. Informal negotiations were taking place all the time (for example, the receptionists started to make Washington his coffee in return for no complaint from him if they added extra patients to his surgery list).

However, it became clear that when I returned, he and I would have to negotiate formally over other changes. Because several key team members left anyway, a new situation was, once again, inevitable. A very small organisation is relatively insecure and personnel are not necessarily easily replaced.

The negotiations
In summary, I conceded on the formality of PHCT meetings. They became more structured and occurred only once a week. I accepted the need for some protocols and rules. The changeover of community staff and the new practice nurse led to a situation where more explicit statements of policy and practice were necessary. I agreed to greater supervision of some of the jobs, for example the ante-natal clinic became entirely shared, and the midwives lost some of their autonomy. He conceded other elements of control, agreeing for example to relative autonomy for the community psychiatric nurse and district nurses. He recognised the manager's role and the importance of Georgia's jobs and the discretion she had in carrying them out. (He had to as she threatened to leave!) The true team spirit of the PHCT was lost. These things are so difficult to build and so easy to lose. However, further progress was gained. The first PHCT was overly dependent on its members and the *Theory Y* leadership. The second version was more robust and coped better with personnel changes. The effectiveness of the system was, by reference to the primary purpose, unimpaired. Income from the practice continued to rise.

The impact that the system had in terms of the mission is harder to judge. The local population had certainly greeted the changes very warmly. My analysis of the resistance to change looked suspect in retrospect. The local (presumed parochial) population were simply ignorant of the possibilities. Given the opportunity to take part in the experiment they were very supportive and appreciative. The new systems were able to respond to their subsequent ideas and demands. For example, we continued at least one daily 'open' surgery in parallel with appointments; starting no smoking classes; we set up genuine well-women clinics run by female staff only.

An evaluation

> 'The stone that is rolling can gather no moss;
> For master and servant oft changing is loss.'
>
> Thomas Tusser

As a system, we should ask if the model in this practice proved to be efficient and effective. Efficiency is classically the ratio of inputs to outputs. It is difficult to weigh up the end result after five years of change. Certainly more patients were going through the system. The practice size had increased from less than 2,000 to over 2,500. Individual patients were making vastly increased use of the system. It is beyond the scope of this account to measure the relative ratio of well patients out to ill patients in; but certain proxy measures are available. For example, the high vaccination uptake, the uptake of smears amongst women at risk, the less than average prescribing costs, etc. The reputation of the practice was also improved. The amount of money required to make the system work was, however, also vastly increased. Many of my original objectives were met. The practice was making much more use of individual expertise. Colleagues were enjoying their jobs more, and I had successfully delegated many tasks to the team members. The infrastructure was transformed. Efficient new subsystems, like practice management and record keeping (and many other information tasks) were added to the practice. The first model of a PHCT was not sustained. I think there were some design faults (too much insularity) and some process faults (decision taking and role accountability were inefficiently democratic – it was fun – but we spent a lot of time talking about things rather than doing things), but in the end its demise owed a lot to the extreme bad luck of my sick leave.

The second model of a PHCT was less democratic but probably stronger. In the final analysis it was strong enough to withstand further changes. The new General Practitioner's contract in April 1990 was met and coped with almost without a ripple of stress, partly because many of its demands were already common practice for the PHCT. I had myself become dispensable and left almost exactly five years after I had arrived.

Conclusion

'We for a certainty are not the first
Have sat in taverns while the tempest hurled
Their hopeful plans to emptiness, and cursed
Whatever brute and blackguard made this world.'

A E Housman

The sick leave I have referred to made me unhappy for a long time. As it occurred as a result of my work and subsequently appeared to be instrumental in destroying what I had been helping to build, I blamed the incident for the 'bereavement' I suffered at the loss of the team I had so much enjoyed being part of. I have defined general practice as an open system designed to transform ill or distressed patients into well and confident people; a system which is ideal when the subsystems cooperate in a democratic, collective way to achieve their shared goals (the mission and the primary purpose). I have described progress towards this ideal via two models of a PHCT. The first emerged directly from a plan, the second as a result of formal and informal negotiations between the players. Irrespective of the failure of the first model, the end result was a success; it met the requirements of the system definition. Albeit the PHCT was integrated by standardisation rather than according to the original plan, the negotiated order within the final organisation (recognising that it remains in a state of constant change, this account merely ends at the time I left) made it much stronger.

PART III

Conclusions

Conclusions

Issues in front-line management in the NHS

Can we draw any general conclusions from our ten Case Studies about the characteristics of front-line organisations in the NHS and the nature of the challenges that they pose to doctors as their managers? Clearly, our sample of these units is neither large in size nor truly random in the way that it was selected. In addition, the Case Studies have all been written by participants who later chose a career in public health medicine and might be seen as sharing an atypically critical view of specialities which they did not make their own. Nevertheless, while it is necessary to be tentative and cautious in making generalisations from the descriptions, there are at least prima-facie grounds for believing that in many ways these Case Studies represent much contemporary practice. The ten cases were selected from a much larger corpus of projects completed by students over several years and are typical of them. Furthermore, the nature of the issues identified in the studies have been widely discussed with colleagues working in different parts of the NHS who have confirmed their relevance to their own experiences and have often gone on to offer similar examples of management practice which they have encountered themselves. Perhaps even more to the point, we believe that it can be shown that the organisational and professional cultures which help explain the issues raised by the Case Studies, are not peculiar to their particular circumstances, but are encountered across the NHS as a whole.

In this concluding chapter we revisit the Case Studies to explore what they have to say about the nature of front-line units in the NHS both in terms of their formal structure and their behavioural characteristics. This leads us to a brief consideration of these units as small-scale social systems and the importance for doctors as managers of being able to understand and respond to them as such. Factors explaining the failure of many doctors in front-line management positions to develop these skills are examined. The remaining part of the chapter addresses ways in which the effectiveness of doctors as managers might be enhanced. For doctors already in posts as managers we outline a series of steps by which they can begin the analysis of the units they lead and consider ways of responding to issues of the kind we have raised in this study. Looking to future generations of doctors, we discuss ways in which their selection and training can be adapted to take full account of their destined roles as managers.

Some key characteristics of front-line units

Formal structure. Nearly all the front-line units described in this book share the common characteristic of multi-disciplinary staffing, and the dominance of hierarchy in their formal lines of command. In addition, in the units located in hospitals it is normal to find dual or triple functions – with training and, sometimes, research being added to the goal of treatment. The result is that, in spite in several cases of being quite small in scale, the structure of most of the units is relatively complex.

Multi-disciplinary structures in the hospital front-line units described in this book combine separately managed medical and nursing hierarchies, but also rely on the support of other staff groups for technical, catering, maintenance and cleaning services. In general practice, the management of practice staff is integrated under the partners but community nurses working with the practice come under the separate management of the district health authority (or, increasingly, a local health service trust) and social workers, whether formally attached to the practice or not, are employed by the local social services department. Some of the specific issues in working in a multi-disciplinary context have been clearly depicted in the Case Studies, as in the relationships between hospital doctors and nurses (Case Studies 1, 2, and 7), and between general practitioners and community nurses and other staff (Case Studies 8 and 10). All of these examples illustrated the nature of the challenges of building working relationships across hierarchical systems where there is no one person in undisputed control of the whole operation.

Establishing such working links can be complicated, as some of the Case Studies also suggest (eg Case Studies 1, 4, and 7), by the nature of the individual hierarchies themselves. Conventionally, the medical and. nursing professions have developed very clear command structures which have tended to be seen as justifying authoritative decision making. In the hospital, this situation derives both from the fact that the consultants heading the different 'firms', as we have shown in the Introduction, are the only doctors with permanent positions in the organisation, and from their professional status as the most expert practitioners in the teams.

The nursing hierarchy, particularly in hospitals, is still a prevalent and separate influence but can be seen as reinforcing authoritative views of management. Its origins lie in the post-Florence Nightingale era of the mid-to-late nineteenth century. The profession's hierarchical traditions have been drawn from the army, religious orders and girls' public schools. The discipline characteristic of nursing organisation was reinforced, until recent times, by the fact that most nurses lived in nursing homes which were subject to that same hierarchy (Abel-Smith, 1960).

In general practice, as the Case Studies show, the relationship between doctors as partners is more commonly one of equality or collegiality. However, in relating to other professional groups such as community nurses, they may well adopt more hierarchical attitudes learned in their hospital-based training. A further complicating factor, in the Case Studies located in hospitals, is the multiple goals of many front-line units. It has been shown (Case Studies 2, 4, 5, and 7) how the training of doctors and nurses is an integral part of many of these micro-organisations. Further, in some settings, research is added as a major (Case Study 4), or minor (Case Study 2) goal.

In sum, these features of the formal structures and functions of front-line NHS units present a picture of relatively complex organisations which can be much more difficult to manage effectively than their size alone would suggest. Moreover, the complexity is increased by the infinite variation in the patients entering the organisations with respect to, not only their manifest clinical conditions, but their behavioural character-istics. In these circumstances, the importance for managers to have a good understanding of the behavioural characteristics of the units themselves is evident.

Behavioural characteristics. The front-line units described in this book all, without exception, contained a significant element of informal organisa-tion beneath the surface of the formal structure. Put another way, each of them had a latent or hidden organisation in addition to its manifest organisation. We have seen, for example, how people in relatively low level posts in terms of the prevailing formal hierarchies can have a disproportionate influence on the nature of the running of a unit (eg *Sister B* in Case Study 1, the Higher Clerical Officer (HCO) in Case Study 3, the SHOs in Case Study 5). It has also been shown how informal negotiations can be vital to the effective operation of routine activities such as the management of an operating theatre (Case Study 2) or a general practice (Case Studies 8, 9 and 10).

To understand the origins of such latent organisations and the ways in which they function and then to manage them effectively, it is necessary, we suggest, to be able to analyse their internal workings as miniature social systems. More specifically, as an action perspective would imply, this requires the capacity to understand the perspectives and motivation of the different members of the unit and others it works with and through, to appreciate the nature of the continuing negotiations between these actors and how they relate to stability and change in the activities of the unit.

The Case Studies as social systems: negotiations, conflict and leadership

If the cases presented in this book are re-visited from such a perspective, it is relatively easy to separate out those units where a negotiated order had evolved which appeared to be defined favourably by the main actors involved, from those where this had not been achieved. It is also possible to identify some of the consequences of either situation for these actors and, in some cases, to assess the likely consequences for patients.

Case Studies 1, 2, and 10 describe negotiated orders in an acute surgery unit, an operating theatre, and a general practice where a working relationship was established which was apparently supported by all the principal actors. Case Studies 4 and 8 describe situations which began with, or moved into conflict but later evolved into negotiated orders more acceptable to the different interest groups within the organisation. In all these cases individuals can be identified who played key roles in developing or maintaining the negotiated order. Interestingly, in only two of the five cases were the most senior managers in the unit amongst these individuals and both of these were in general practices (Case Studies 8 and 10). In Case Study 1, the central figure in the development of the quasi-participative system which constituted the latent organisation was one of the Sisters. In Case Study 2, the smooth working of the operating theatre seems to have resulted from the informal collaboration and mutual understanding of several of the permanent members of the team. In Case Study 4 relationships within the unit were rescued from disaster by a perceptive Registrar who deliberately set about constructing a more viable and rewarding working environment for the junior members of the firm. In all of these examples it would appear that the working relationships supported by the negotiated order would be likely to serve patient and staff interests in that they acted to maintain the smooth running of a service, or were an essential ingredient in restoring or developing such a service. It can also be seen that in all of these examples at the heart of the negotiated order was the concept of the unit as a team, sharing not only common treatment goals but also in satisfying other important needs of all its members. In most cases this involved a significant element of consultation or participation.

In contrast, four of the Case Studies describe situations where some of the key interest groups were excluded from the negotiated order, or where the position was more accurately described as one of conflict than order. In the school health clinic (Case Study 3) the Higher Clerical Officer (HCO) and the Senior Clinical Medical Officer (SCMO) formed a dominant coalition which virtually excluded the main body of CMOs from

160

all involvement in the organisation apart from carrying out their own immediate duties. The system worked because of the low expectations of the CMOs, but was vulnerable in that when the HCO was away no one could deputise for her and patients requiring specialist assessment remained unallocated. In Case Studies 4, 5 and 7 the junior doctors were excluded from management decisions. In all cases their training was adversely affected. In Case Study 4, the research task was put in jeopardy and relations with patients' GPs put at risk. In Case Study 5 the failure to devise an acceptable rota led to periods when both night and week-end cover in the hospital were perilously overstretched. In Case Study 7 the powerful dominant coalition of midwives, by their treatment of the junior doctors, restricted their learning and turned them off careers in obstetrics and, by freezing out the new midwife recruited to introduce modern methods into the unit, protected conservative practice.

These units were characterised by hierarchical relationships unmodified by notions of the unit as a team (although in Case Study 4 a team approach was eventually imported). Neither consultative nor participative practice was evident and the result for the junior staff concerned was either conflict or withdrawal, and for patients the risk or reality of a less effective service.

Case Studies 6 and 9 describe situations in which the managerial leadership of the units concerned was challenged, and eventually a shift of power was achieved in episodes that seem to have been personally stressful and costly for a number of the people involved. In the first case, the issues in the Paediatric Unit were fought out at the informal level, only surfacing to be openly confronted after several years, and when a significant change in power relationships had already taken place. In the second a successful attempt was made to get the whole medical partnership to agree to the construction of a new surgery but the same effort was apparently not put into sustaining support and involvement throughout the change process itself. The result was an outcome adversely affecting the health and commitment of some of the doctors, and damaging to the coherence of the team as a whole.

Some implications for doctors as front-line managers

Perhaps the most salient message to emerge from this review is that the behavioural aspects of organisation of front-line units in the NHS are much too important to leave to chance and far too complex to respond to simplistic top-down management. As in most organisations where professionals occupy the main hands-on roles and are expected and required to exercise considerable discretion in doing their work, management must win both their commitment and their cooperation if it is to achieve the effectiveness, efficiency and economy that it is constantly urged to pursue.

The rewards for achieving such involvement, however, are considerable. If ever the circumstances existed for achieving synergy in human organisation – where the satisfaction of individual and organisational needs are brought into harmony, health care must provide one of the best opportunities to do so. The health care professions attract a high proportion of staff with a moral, rather than merely instrumental, commitment to their work. The units of service delivery are small enough and have sufficient autonomy to allow the evolution of management arrangements which maximise the expression of this commitment. It is difficult to see how an accurate picture of the conditions needed to plan for such developments can be achieved, without, as a minimum, extensive consultation with all the main groups of staff involved. In the longer run, a framework for participation in all significant decisions affecting the unit may well be implied.

If these are reasonable conclusions to draw from a review of the experience of our Case Studies, why are such practices far from being the common way of managing front-line units in the NHS? And when these practices do emerge, at least in the Case Studies, why is it apparently as much a matter of luck as leadership – or leadership from unofficial leaders as often as from the formally appointed managers? The answers to these questions would seem to lie in a cluster of factors affecting the attitudes, recruitment, training, and career paths of doctors, and their working environments, which taken together, may account for a kind of blindness or indifference to the key behavioural elements in management.

Doctors and the roots of a managerial malaise

A logical starting point for examining the origins of prevailing attitudes in the medical profession is to consider its main sources of recruitment. Entry to the profession has been dominated in the post-war years by the middle classes (Wilding, 1982). As a high status profession it has a disproportionate intake from the public schools and as a result has been subject to the traditional authority values and relationships that tend to typify such establishments. Translated into leadership these influences are likely to encourage an authoritative style and scepticism about the need for more behavioural approaches in management.

Once entrenched in a well-established profession, such values and practices are difficult to displace since entry, training and promotion are largely controlled by the profession itself (Goode, 1957). In medicine,

162

consultants, through their influence on recruitment to medical schools and on selection committees for the promotion of doctors to consultant rank, have a major role in these processes and through them the reproduction of the profession. Interestingly, however, the GPs in the Case Studies seem more aware of management as an issue than the hospital consultants. This is probably due to the selection of particular kinds of doctors into general practice on the basis of their greater interest in relationships and the fact that practices also operate as small businesses in themselves.

The restricted nature of the main career paths open to doctors, which we noted in the Introduction, and the criteria on which they are promoted, are further factors contributing to the low status of managerial skills in the profession. Most medical careers lead either to an appointment as a hospital consultant or a principal in general practice, both of which types of post almost inevitably involve managerial responsibilities. However, promotion to these posts is mainly determined by professional ability, assessed primarily by other consultants and managerial competence plays little or no part in the process.

These various influences reinforcing traditional, authoritative views of leadership and inhibiting the development of more open and informed approaches to the challenges of front-line management are supported by the character of relationships with the other two main actors in the medical arena, the nurse and the patient. The nursing profession has in many ways modelled itself on the medical profession and developed a comparable hierarchical structure and similar traditional authority values (Ackroyd, 1992). Patients in a health service free at the point of consumption, and in a society that itself is still remarkably class ridden, have tended to exhibit deferential and uncritical attitudes to their doctors. In these ways both nurses and patients tend to underpin rather than undermine the status quo.

These various factors may go some way to explain the weaknesses of doctors as front-line managers implied in several of the Case Studies, and their ability to resist change in spite of such failings. However, it may now be asked whether the wider changes currently taking place in the NHS leading towards a more managerial culture will at last provide a real challenge to the profession to develop more effective front-line leadership.

The new NHS and managerial culture

On the face of it, the greater emphasis placed on management following Griffiths, and again in the development of the internal market might have been expected to sharpen the focus on the management of the front-line unit. If it has done so, however, it would seem mainly in terms of measurement and control rather than the behavioural dynamics of such units. In other words, it would seem that the issue of compliance continues to be seen as unproblematic or as being simply a question of asserting authority backed by sufficient sanctions. Dyson, (1984) identified the general management proposals in the Griffiths report as being rather ineffectual in the absence of limited tenure consultant contracts. He argued that only when such contracts prevailed, and were only renewable after clinical performance had been assessed in relation to resources used, could general managers achieve change.

On the other hand, he also believed that the use of such powers would cause long and divisive conflict with the medical profession. To date, short-term contracts and performance-related pay have been restricted to general managers and not extended to medical staff.

Nevertheless, the District General Manager or Chief Executive of a hospital trust now has the right to sit in on consultant appointment committees rather than just attend as an observer as in the past. Furthermore, tightly drawn job descriptions which include budgetary and other management responsibilities are reviewed annually for each consultant (Working for Patients, 1989). Although not yet used in practice, it is now legitimate for hospital trusts to appoint new consultants on short-term contracts. In the changed NHS so far, however, it appears unlikely that the greater power of general management will be used to promote the development of behavioural skills in health service management. The dominant culture remains one of performance indicators, standards and target setting rather than a concern with how to get there.

The main lesson of this book, however, is that such an approach which takes no account of the complex factors affecting people's motivation and commitment, nor of their willingness and ability to work together in a particular context, is a recipe for creating disaffection, alienation and underperformance. Doctors, who readily respect the importance of knowledge in their own field of medicine, need to seek a similar understanding in the field of behaviour in organisations if they are to create the conditions for effective front-line management in health care. Further, in the current climate it seems that the initiative for such a development cannot be expected to emerge from the business managers of the NHS and, in spite of the impediments in tradition and practice we have described, will have to come from amongst the doctors themselves.

Some practical steps for doctors as managers in the analysis of front-line organisations

The behavioural sciences offer the beginner none of the relative certainties which characterise the first steps in the natural sciences. The contested nature of 'reality' becomes immediately apparent in organisational studies as soon as the different perspectives of different interest groups are considered. Yet, as we have suggested in the Introduction, there are sufficient areas of common ground to make social analysis a worthwhile venture. The ten point check-list listed below is offered as a starting point for doctors as front-line managers who want to explore behavioural aspects of the units they lead and to review their own roles as managers in the light of the exercise. Those who find the experience useful may also find the literature referred to in the Introduction a helpful way into a fuller understanding of the concepts underlying the points below.

1. What kind of an organisation are you managing?
The contingency approach to organisational analysis has shown the importance of distinguishing between different types of organisation related to differences in the tasks they are carrying out and the implications these have for controlling them. Thus routine, machine-like processes may call for different management structures from those concerned with flexible, tailor-made responses to dissimilar situations. Where is your unit located, for example, on a continuum between the most mechanistic and most organic definitions of the work task? Or, taking the Mintzberg typology of organisations outlined in the Introduction (pages 21–3), which of his main configurations comes closest to describing the nature of your unit? Or would it more appropriately be described as a hybrid combining elements of more than one of these?

2. What is the scope and nature of your authority as a manager?
We have seen in the Case Studies that the interdisciplinary nature of many front-line units may mean that the formal or legitimate authority of the doctors is often more limited than their acknowledged professional seniority might suggest. It is important for doctors, as managers, to be able to distinguish between the different bases for power and influence and to be able to assess accurately the nature of the basis for their own leadership in shaping their managerial strategies.

3. What goals are you pursuing?
Clarity about goals is an essential prerequisite of effective management.

Drawing on systems theory, it has been suggested in this book that it is important to begin by identifying the primary task that your part of the organisation must fulfil in order to survive. Our Case Studies have suggested that where this task is well understood it usually attracts the support of most members of the unit, whatever their general attitudes to the leadership. But survival has both a short-run and long-run dimension. We have seen how failure to give due attention to the long-run was fatal to one unit (Case Study 1) and how, when junior staff were alienated by their seniors, they exhibited no concern for the longer-term future of the institution in which they were being trained (Case Study 5). Most organisations look to more than mere survival, however, and have secondary or mission tasks. It is important to separate these out clearly from the primary task, not only to ensure a proper prioritising of goals, but also because the different types of task are likely to be perceived differently by other members of the unit and the case for them may need separate justification.

4. What structures exist to achieve the goals of the unit?
A critical evaluation of the appropriateness of the existing organisation, needs to include a close examination of its current structures and processes. Again, a systems approach as outlined in the Introduction (pages 24–6) offers a useful way of doing this. The unit is seen as an 'open system', taking in, for example, patients requiring treatment and the resources required for that treatment; the treatment process itself is the 'conversion' activity, and the treated patient the 'output' of the system. Working out the detail of these stages, together with any subsystems within them, provides a framework for reviewing all the main activities of the unit and their interrelationships. It also encourages you to ask if each of the subsystems has appropriate management. Repeating the operation for secondary or missionary tasks allows you to see how far the different goals you are pursuing, for example, teaching and research, are compatible and if they are not, how the system as a whole might be modified to make them so.

5. Who are the main actors in the organisation you are managing?
At this point it is time to broaden your focus to include the all-important human factors in your analysis. The action perspective briefly outlined in the Introduction (pages 28–9) provides a useful framework for the process. Your first task is to identify the main individuals or groups of individuals who make up the organisation you are managing. In a small unit of a dozen or so people this is easy enough but where numbers are larger it is helpful to use the concept of the 'ideal type' to simplify the process. This involves grouping people who appear to share particular characteristics as, for example, consultants, junior doctors, staff nurses, enrolled nurses,

although these categories may need sub-dividing where there are significant differences within them as in aspects of their motivation to work, their types of commitment and styles of interaction.

6. What is the nature of the commitment to the organisation of the different actors?

The next stage in the analysis is to seek to understand how the actors relate to the organisation. What are their main motives for working in your unit and what is the nature of their commitment to it? In the Introduction we suggested that one useful way of classifying these orientations was in terms of moral, calculative, and alienative attachments but there are, of course, many other ways of classifying motivation.

7. What is your strategy for supporting and motivating the different actors in the unit?

This is essentially a question about your style of leadership. We have seen in this book how in many cases, particularly in hospitals, doctors seem oblivious to the possibility of employing any but an authoritarian method of management. But it has also been demonstrated in the Case Studies, as in the literature, that a whole range of styles exists and how, on occasion, these appear to produce very different results. For a start, try locating your own methods of management on Likert's continuum between Exploitive Authoritative and Participative styles (Introduction, page 27). It can also be helpful in this process to ask your colleagues for a frank assessment of your style – if you can take it!

8. How well does your style of management match the patterns of motivation and commitment of staff in the unit?

Looking back on your review of the motivation of the members of your unit, consider the appropriateness of your leadership style. A largely moral commitment by staff, for instance, suggests a management style that recognises and reinforces that commitment, encouraging a sharing of decisions and responsibilities wherever feasible. A more instrumental commitment might justify a more tightly controlled response. It is often easy to deceive ourselves into thinking that our leadership style is well-perceived by those we lead, since our position of authority is itself likely to shelter us from adverse comment. However, this self-analysis will be useless if we cannot penetrate through such protective screening to construct an accurate picture of how the other actors in the unit see the situation.

9. What is the nature of the negotiated order in your organisation?

The final aim in this exercise is to build a model of the 'real' organisation in the sense of the negotiated relationships which actually deliver its work and the distribution of power that underpins it. In so far as you can make the latent organisation visible you should be able to construct a view of how favourably or unfavourably members of the unit define their work context, and to what extent they are acting to maintain or change it. In terms of every day activities you should have a good idea of the actual operating practices which they have built up between each other, and with others outside the unit, as well as of the nature of the exchanges which sustain them. You will be able to compare this web of relationships with the formal structure of your unit as a system (4. above) and consider to what extent they are in harmony or disharmony. This, in sum, relatively stable or unstable, is the negotiated order through which the unit operates.

10. Analysis as a foundation for development and change.
If this exercise in organisational analysis has been even partially successful you will be well placed to consider the relationship between the organisation you have delineated and the quality of the work it carries out. You should also be in a better position to consider the possibilities of development and change in the unit. Elsewhere, drawing on the literature of the management of change (Forster and Hadley, 1989), we have reviewed some of the key factors related to successful change. These start with an understanding of the forces promoting and resisting change, consider the process of 'unfreezing' an existing equilibrium, introducing the changes, and then of 'refreezing' the new structures and processes. A perceptive analysis of your own organisation should enable you to identify both the promoters and resisters of change and to understand their perspectives. It should also help you to elaborate with them the most acceptable means of introducing change while recognising their needs, and assist you in consolidating the altered structure in ways that are as consistent as possible with the prevailing patterns of motivation and commitment.

Other factors in enhancing the management of front-line units

The evidence of this book, we believe, provides ample grounds for believing that the quality of front-line management in the NHS could be substantially enhanced by improving awareness and understanding of the behavioural dimensions of organisations, and developing leadership skills built on these. The achievement of such changes will, in the end, turn on how far the individual doctor-managers become interested and committed to them. Yet this in turn is likely to be influenced in no small way by the processes of selection for medical training and for subsequent promotion. Finally, the influence of the particular culture of management encouraged

168

at the macro level by government and by NIIS boards from the Department of Health downwards could turn out to be the most decisive factor of all.

Selection

It remains an open question as to how far management skills of the kind we have been concerned with in this book can be taught. It seems likely, at least, that some people have more aptitude for developing them than others. Currently, as far as we are aware, there is no attempt to test for such aptitudes in the selection of medical students and little in the way of screening at later stages in promotion up the ladder to consultant grade or general practitioner. It would seem to us, that at the very least, there is a strong case for introducing some tests of interpersonal skills in the initial selection of medical students and, where later stages of training are concerned, for assessment of both knowledge and practice in this area.

Training

As almost all doctors are likely to end up managing at least small teams, there are good grounds for introducing a required element of training in organisation and management within their undergraduate course. It is not within the scope of this book to attempt to delineate the full compass of such training. We would argue strongly, however, that it should go beyond familiarisation with a range of management techniques to lay the foundations for the acquisition of the skills of organisational analysis. The course from which the Case Studies in this book originated provides one possible example of how this can be achieved. It also illustrates the importance, within any such training, of giving students the opportunity to test out the theories to which they are being exposed on real-life organisations. One possible way of achieving this opportunity in under-graduate medical education would be to introduce the theoretical element of an organisation and management course just before the elective period of training which usually comes in the penultimate clinical training year. The elective placement could then form the subject of the student's organisation project.

We noted earlier that the availability of management training, provided by various bodies for junior doctors, tends to be haphazard rather than systematic. In spite of clinical demands, there is a fundamental need for the continuous exposure of junior doctors, especially including those whose intention it is to continue their careers in front-line units, to a programme of management skills. Whether such programmes could encompass the joint involvement of juniors, consultants and others in analysing the current experience of a clinical firm's management is a moot point. It may prove too threatening, but achieving maximum assimilation of management skills for future use by junior doctors implies that learning

169

is through analysis of real life experiences, even if carried out separately from the team environment. What is most important is that training in management skills is not dominated by the 'business plan' culture of the changed NHS.

The culture of the NHS

It seems unlikely that any of these changes would make much impact unless eventually the culture of the NHS as a whole is supportive of them. The post-Griffiths NHS might, on the face of it, be seen as likely to provide a promising environment for improving the quality of front-line management. The emphasis in Griffiths' own report (1983) on general management opened the way for a fundamental reconsideration of the traditional assumptions underlying NHS administration. The subsequent adoption of the internal market and the development of NHS trusts gives further prominence to the importance of management. So far however, much of the official rhetoric has been about budgets and increasingly tight control, and there has been remarkably little interest in the questions of the kind raised in this book dealing with the internal functioning of front-line units. As a contemporary student of the NHS recently noted, this seems like a particularly retrograde step in the light of evidence that private sector management is moving in the opposite direction:

'In the private sector, radical initiatives are being taken to increase the team-working and cooperative capacities of employees in a situation where they have scarcely existed, whilst, at the very same time, public sector management often works on the assumption that they must achieve exclusive power and control over work perform-ance in the manner assumed to be operative in the private sector'

(Ackroyd, 1992, pp 327–328).

Of course, there are health service managers who realise the importance of cultivating responsive organisations in which there is a substantial devolution of responsibility to well-managed front-line teams (see eg Hadley and Young, 1990, pp 216–222). The question is whether in the future it will come to be recognised that such developments, based on increasing the quality of doctors as managers, are essential in maximising the effectiveness of these teams, and through them the effectiveness of services provided to patients by the NHS as a whole.

References

Abel-Smith, B. (1960) *A History of the Nursing Profession.* London: Heinemann.

Accounting for Health. (1973) Report of a King's Fund Working Party on the application of economic principles to health service management. London: King Edward's Hospital's Fund for London.

Ackroyd, S. (1992) Nurses and the Prospects of Participative Management in Nursing in Soothill, K. et al (eds) *Themes and Perspectives in Nursing.* London: Harper Collins.

Ackroyd, S., Hughes, J. & Soothill, K. (1989) Public Sector Services and their Management. *Journal of Management Studies.* v26, No 6.

British Medical Association (1970) *Report of the Working Party on Primary Medical Care.* Planning Unit Report No. 4. London: BMA.

Burrell, G. & Morgan, G. (1979) *Sociological Paradigms and Organizational Analysis.* London: Heinemann Educational Books.

Butler, G.V. (1986) *Organization and Management.* Englewood Cliffs, N.J.: Prentice-Hall.

Carnall, C.A. (1990) *Managing Change in Organizations.* Englewood Cliffs, New Jersey: Prentice Hall.

Checkland, P. (1981) *Systems Thinking, Systems Practice.* Chichester: Wiley.

Child, J. (1972) Organizational structure, environment and performance: the role of strategic choice, *Sociology,* 6, 1–22.

Coch, L. & French, J. (1948) Overcoming Resistance to Change, *Human Relations,* 1, 4, 525–532.

Committee on Child Health Services. (1976) *Fit for the Future.* (SDM Court, chairman) (Cmnd 6680) London: HMSO.

Cooper, C. & Marshall, J. (1976) Occupational sources of stress: a review of the literature relating to coronary heart disease and mental ill health. *Journal of Occupational Psychology*, 49, 11–28.

Cope, D. (1986) *Organisation Development and Action Research in Hospitals* Aldershot: Gower.

Cox, D. (1991) Health service management – a sociological view: Griffiths and the non-negotiated order of the hospital in Gabe, J. et al (eds) *The Sociology of the Health Service*. London: Routledge.

Dalton, M. (1959) *Men Who Manage* New York: John Wiley.

Dalton, G.W., Barnes, L.B., & Zaleznik, A. (1968) *The distribution of authority in formal organisations.* Harvard University, Boston.

Department of Health. (1990) *The Quality of Medical Care:* Report of the Standing Medical Advisory Committee. London: HMSO.

Department of Health and Social Security. (1972) *Management Arrangements for the Reorganised National Health Service.* London: HMSO.

Department of Health and Social Security. (1972) *Second Report of the Joint Working Party on the Organisation of the Medical Work in Hospitals.* London: HMSO.

Department of Health and Social Security. (1974) *Third Report of the Joint Working Party on the Organisation of the Medical Work in Hospitals.* London: HMSO.

Department of Health and Social Security. (1983) *NHS Management Inquiry* (The Griffiths Report) DA(83)38 London.

Department of Health and the Welsh Office. (1989) *General Practice in the National Health Service: A New Contract.* London.

Dillner, L. (1993) Hospitals running out of cash. *British Medical Journal.* 306, 355.

Donabedian, A. (1966) Evaluating the quality of medical care. *Milbank Memorial Fund Quarterly*, 44: Suppl 166–206.

Drummond, M.F. Stoddart, G.L. & Torrance, G.W. (1987) *Methods for the Economic Evaluation of Health Care Programmes.* Oxford: Oxford University Press.

Dyson, R. (1984) Griffiths inquiry: a personal perspective. *British Medical Journal*, 288, 255–257.

Etzioni, A. (1961) *A Comparative Analysis of Complex Organizations*. New York: Free Press.

Flagle, C.D. (1962) Operations Research in the Health Services. *Operations Research*, 10: 591–603.

Flynn, R. (1992) *Structures of Control in Health Management*. London: Routledge.

Forster, D.P & Hadley, R. (1989) The NHS Reforms: Conditions for Successful Change? *Health Services Management*, 85, 215–218.

French, J.R.P. & Raven, B. (1970) The Bases of Social Power in D. Cartwright and A. Zander (eds) *Group Dynamics*. New York: Harper and Row.

Fromm, E. (1956) *The Sane Society*. London: Routledge and Kegan Paul.

Fry, J. (1988) *General practice and primary health care: 1940s–1980s*. Nuffield Provincial Hospitals Trust, London.

Garmarnikow, E. (1978) Sexual Division of labour: the case of nursing. In *Feminism and Materialism* (Kuhn A. & Wolfe A., Eds). London: Routledge & Kegan Paul.

General Medical Council: Education Committee. (1980) *Recommendations on Basic Medical Education*, London.

Goldthorpe, J. et al (1968) *The Affluent Worker: Industrial Attitudes and Behaviour*. Cambridge: Cambridge University Press.

Goode, W.J. (1957) Community within a community: the professions. *American Sociological Review* 22, 194–200.

Gouldner, A.W. (1954) *Patterns of Industrial Bureaucracy*. Glencoe, Ill.: Free Press.

Hadley, R. & Young, K. (1990) *Creating a Responsive Public Service*. London: Harvester–Wheatsheaf.

Ham, C. (1991) *The New National Health Service*. Oxford: Radcliffe Medical Press.

Hampton, J. (1983) *The End of Clinical Freedom. British Medical Journal*, 287, 1237–8.

Handy, C.B. (1985) *Understanding Organizations*. Harmondsworth: Penguin.

Haywood, S. Alaszewski, A. (1980) *Crisis in the Health Service: the politics of management*. Croom Helm, London: 1980.

Hoffenburg, R. (1987) *Clinical Freedom*. London: Nuffield Provincial Hospitals Trust.

Holmes, T.H. & Rahe, R.H. (1967) The social readjustment rating scale. *Journal of Psychosomatic Research*. 11, 213–218.

Homans, G. (1951) *The Human Group*. London: Routledge Kegan Paul.

Hopkins, R. (1987) Doctors as general managers: To be or not to be. *British Medical Journal*, 295, 1360–1361.

Hughes, D. (1988) When nurse knows best: some aspects of nurse/doctor interaction in a casualty department. *Sociology of Health & Illness*, 10; 1–22.

Jee, M. & Reason, L. (1988) *Action on stress at work*. London: Health Education Authority.

Joint Committee on Higher Medical Training. (1991) *Training Handbook 1990/91*. London. (Mimeo)

Kanter, R.M. (1983) *The Change Masters*. London: Allen and Unwin.

Kanter, R.M. (1992) *The Challenge of Organizational Change*. New York: Free Press.

Kast, F.E. & Rosenzweig, J.E. (1985) *Organization and Management: A Systems and Contingency Approach*. New York: McGraw-Hill (4th edition).

Kearns, D. (1976) *Lyndon Johnson and the American Dream*. London: Andre Deutsch.

Kotter, J. P. (1978) *Organizational Dynamics*. Reading, Mass.: Addison-Wesley.

Kotter, J. & Schlesinger, L. (1979) 'Choosing Strategies for Change', *Harvard Business Review*, 57, 2, 106–14.

Levitt, R. & Wall, A. (1984) *The Reorganised National Health Service*. Croom Helm: London.

Lewin, K. (1947) Group decision and social change. in *Readings in Social Psychology*. Eds. Newcomb T.M. and Hartley E.L. New York: Holt Rinehart and Winston.

Likert, R. (1967) *The Human Organization*. New York: McGraw-Hill.

Lupton, T. (1963) *On the Shop Floor*. Oxford: Pergamon.

Mackay, L. (1989) *Nursing a Problem*. Milton Keynes: Open University.

Mackay, L. (1993) *Conflicts in Care*. London: Chapman Hall.

Maccoby, M. (1988) *Why Work: Motivating and Leading the New Generation*. New York: Simon and Schuster.

McGregor, D. (1960) *The Human Side of Enterprise*. New York: McGraw-Hill.

Maslow, A.H. (1954) *Motivation and Personality*. New York: Harper Bros.

Maslow, A.H. (1965) *Eupsychian Management*. Homewood, Ill.: Richard Irwin and The Dorsey Press.

Mayo, E. (1933) *The Human Problems of an Industrial Civilization*. New York: MacMillan.

Mechanic, D. (1962) Sources of Power of Lower Participants in Complex Organizations, *Administrative Science Quarterly*. 7, 3, 349–64.

Miller, E.J. and Rice, A.K. (1967) *Systems of Organisation: the Control of Task and Sentient Boundaries*. London: Tavistock.

Ministry of Health. (1967) *First Report of the Joint Working Party on the Organisation of the Medical Work in Hospitals*. London: HMSO.

Ministry of Health and Scottish Home and Health Department. (1966) *Report of the Committee on Senior Nursing Staff Structure* (Chairman B Salmon). London: HMSO.

Mintzberg, H. (1979) *The Structuring of Organizations*. Englewood Cliffs, New Jersey: Prentice-Hall.

Mintzberg, H. (1989) *Mintzberg on Management*. New York: The Free Press.

Mumford, P. (1989) Doctors in the driving seat. *The Health Service Journal*, 99, 612–613.

National Health Service Bill. (1946) (Cmnd 6761) London: HMSO.

National Health Service Reorganisation: England. (1972) (Cmnd. 5055) London: HMSO.

NHS Management Executive. (1991) *Junior Doctors: the New Deal*. Enclosure with Executive Letter EL(91)82.

Neuhauser, P.C. (1988) *Tribal Warfare In Organizations*. Grand Rapids, Mich.: Harper Business.

Office of Health Economics (1974) *The NHS Reorganisation*. London.

Peters, T. (1987) *Thriving on Chaos*. New York: Knopf.

Peters T.J. & Waterman R.H. (1982) *In search of excellence*. New York: Harper & Row.

Pettigrew, A.M. (1973) *The Politics of Organizational Decision-Making*. London: Tavistock.

Porter, S. (1991) A participant observation study of power relations between nurses and doctors in a general hospital. *Journal of Advanced Nursing*, 16; 728–735.

Reed, M. (1985) *Redirections in Organizational Analysis*, London: Tavistock.

Reed, M. and Hughes, M. (eds) (1993) *Rethinking Organization*. London: Sage.

Report by Sir William Beveridge. (1942) *Social Insurance and Allied Services*. (Cmnd 6404) London: HMSO.

Rice, A. K. (1960) *The Enterprise and its Environment: A Systems Theory of Management Organisation*. London: Tavistock.

Roethlisberger, F.J. and Dickson, W.J. (1939) *Management and the Worker*. Cambridge, Mass.: Harvard University Press.

Rogers, C.R. (1972) A Humanistic Conception of Man in J.F. Glass and J.R. Staude (eds) *Humanistic Society*. Pacific Palisades, Cal.: Goodyear.

Royal College of Physicians of London. (1988) *General Professional Training*. London. (Mimeo)

Schein, E.H. (1980) *Organizational Psychology*. Englewood Cliff, N.J.: Prentice Hall, 3rd edition.

Secretaries of State for Health, Wales, Northern Ireland and Scotland. (1989) *Working for Patients*. (Cmnd 555) HMSO, London.

Silverman, D. (1970) *The Theory of Organisations*. London: Heinemann Educational Books.

Strauss, A. et al (1971) The Hospital and its Negotiated Order in F.G. Castles et al (eds) *Decisions, Organizations and Society*. Harmondsworth: Penguin.

Taylor, F.W. (1947) *Scientific Management*. London: Harper and Row.

The Guardian (1987) Doctors resist 'undermining' by managers, 30th June.

Trist, E.L. & Bamforth, K.W. (1951) Some Social and Psychological Consequences of the Longwall Method of Coal Getting, *Human Relations*, 4, 3–38.

von Bertalanffy, L. (1950) An outline of general system theory. *British J Philos Sci*, 1, 134–165.

Watson, B. (1982) Counter-Planning on the Shop Floor in P.J. Frost et al *Organizational Reality: Reports from the Firing Line*. Glenview, Ill.: Scott, Foreman and Company pp. 286–294.

Weber, M. (1947) *The Theory of Economic and Social Organization*. New York: The Free Press.

Wilding, P. (1982) *Professional Power and Social Welfare*. London: Routledge.

Willcocks, A. J. (1967) *The Origins of the National Health Service*. London: Routledge Kegan Paul.

Working for Patients. (1989) *NHS Consultants: Appointments, Contracts and Distinction Awards*. Working Paper 7. London: Department of Health.

Index